well journal

A 12-WEEK GUIDE TO WELLNESS

ISBN: 978-0-9980376-0-8
Copyright © 2019 Jennifer Anthony
All rights reserved.
No portion of this journal may be replicated without permission.

NAME: _____

EMAIL: _____

STARTING DATE: _____

STARTING WEIGHT: _____

GOAL WEIGHT: _____

END WEIGHT: _____

END DATE: _____

How to get the most out of this journal

Making changes to your nutrition, fitness, and lifestyle is a journey of mindfulness that starts with building awareness and a connection to how different choices impact your body.

To help you build this awareness, I created this 12-week journal to give you all the tools to stay organized, plan ahead, set goals, and make connections between your habits and how they impact your body, mind, and spirit.

To get the most out of this journal, here are a few of my top tips for getting the maximum benefit out of each section.

WEEKLY AFFIRMATIONS

Each week will start with a powerful affirmation to help anchor your intentions for the week. Recite these to yourself often to help you stay grounded and connected to your goals!

WEEKLY GOAL SETTING & MEAL PLANNING PAGES

At the beginning of each week you will find goal setting and meal planning pages to help you get organized. I highly advise choosing a regular day of the week (possibly Sunday or Monday) to sit down and map out your goals, meal plan, and grocery list for the next seven days.

GOALS FOR THE WEEK
Use this space to help you focus on your most important goals for the coming week. If you could accomplish just THREE things that would make the biggest impact on your productivity/long term ambitions/stress levels, whether wellness or personal or work related; what would they be? Write them down.

EXERCISE PLAN

The most commonly cited reason why many people don't exercise is because they "don't have time." However, we all have little chunks of time to fit fitness into our day if we plan ahead and act strategically! Look at your calendar and plan what type of exercise you will do this week and what days and what times you have available. Write your plan down and commit to it. If you use another calendar, put your workouts in there too!

NOTE — Don't discount the power of fitting in small chunks of fitness into your day! A 15-minute walk will certainly serve you better than no walk at all.

LOOKING TO ADD A DONE-FOR-YOU FITNESS PLAN TO YOUR ROUTINE? Head on over to coachingbyjennifer.com to find out more about my online fitness programs.

MEAL PLAN & GROCERY LIST

Planning is the key to success when it comes to eating well. Having a plan of what you are going to eat over the course of the week will help you grocery shop, do some food prep, and make your whole week flow more smoothly. Use this page to map out your week.

BONUS TIP — Use a pencil while planning just in case you need to make changes!

DAILY NUTRITION & LIFESTYLE PAGES

For each day of your 12-week journal, you will find a two-page spread to track your food and water intake, fitness and daily step count, daily reflections on how you are feeling, self-care practices, and goal setting.

NUTRITION TRACKER

Track the timing, content, portion sizes, and ingredients of your meals. Check in to make sure you are getting nutrients from each nutritional category listed throughout the day with the nutrition tracker portion of your journal.

If weight loss is your goal, you'll also see a spot on the bottom right hand corner to track your daily steps, weight, and body fat percentage. These are placed to make it easy for you to flip through the pages to see your progress on a day-to-day basis at a glance.

LOOKING FOR PERSONALIZED NUTRITION SUPPORT?
Reach out to me for more information on my one-on-one health coaching programs at coachingbyjennifer.com.

AM REFLECTION - WHAT WOULD MAKE TODAY GREAT?
Jumpstart your morning with this short exercise to help remind yourself of your daily goals and focus on where you can direct your positive energy each day.

WHAT WOULD MAKE TODAY GREAT?
Examples...
1)...call a family member or loved one
2)...make a superfood smoothie for my afternoon snack
3)...go for a walk instead of watching Netflix after dinner

PM GRATITUDE - 3 THINGS I'M GRATEFUL FOR
Before you go to bed each night, take a moment to write down three things you are grateful for each day. Gratitude is scientifically proven to help improve self-esteem, improve psychological and physical health, and even help you sleep better. These reflections are also wonderful to look back at later to help you remember the small and precious positive details of your life.

3 THINGS I'M GRATEFUL FOR
Examples:
1)...the energy I am feeling in the afternoons now that I am eating more nutritious foods
2)...the nice thank you note my sister sent me in the mail
3)...the beautiful sunset I witnessed on my evening walk

ONE THING I WOULD LIKE TO KEEP WORKING ON...
We all have days where we didn't follow through on all our goals. Instead of beating yourself up with a laundry list of things that you "didn't do," try to focus your thoughts on one positive change you would like to make the next day and think about how you might be able to set yourself up for success to follow through with it.

NOTE Don't forget to pat yourself on the back for all the positive steps you **DID** take each day!

IN THE BACK OF THIS JOURNAL

In the back of this journal you will find a few more resources to help you monitor your body transformation progress. Use these tools to help you see the big picture of how the lifestyle changes you are making impact your body and health.

WEIGHT TRACKER
See all of your weight loss and body fat percentage progress at a glance by listing all your weigh-ins in one place. Remember, the scale is not the only sign of progress and certainly not a measure of your self-worth. Use this simply as a progress measuring tool!

BODY MEASUREMENTS
As many have experienced when changing their diet and exercise routines, the scale never tells the whole story. Especially when exercising and building strength, it is completely normal to lose lots of inches around your body and look and feel completely different without seeing a significant change on the scale. I highly recommend you take body measurements at the beginning of your 12-week journey and then again every 2 weeks, recording your body measurement progress on these pages.

BONUS TIP — Take progress photos of yourself from both a front and side profile. These can be a powerful reference point to see progress.

WEEKLY NOTES + FAVORITE MEALS
Have a conversation with your coach or trainer that had you needing to jot down lots of "a-ha!" moments? Come across a lunch idea or recipe you want to remember? Use this space for any notes or reflections you want to keep track of.

MAKE THIS JOURNAL YOUR OWN
I hope you will use this journal to help support your growth and journey towards a healthier and more mindful you. Make it your own and I promise you will come to love the daily practice of reflection that journaling will provide you.

xx jennifer

share your well journal journey!

I WOULD LOVE TO SEE HOW YOU ARE USING THIS JOURNAL
TO HELP YOU LIVE YOUR BEST LIFE.

SHARE A PHOTO OF YOUR JOURNAL ON INSTAGRAM!
TAG ME @COACHINGBYJENNIFER
AND USE THE HASHTAG #WELLJOURNAL.

CHEERS TO YOUR JOURNEY!

Jennifer Lesyna Anthony
Certified Integrative Health Coach & Personal Trainer
Coaching by Jennifer | coachingbyjennifer.com

I AM...

FOCUSED

> "THE CREATION OF A THOUSAND FORESTS
> IS IN ONE ACORN."
> - RALPH WALDO EMERSON

WHAT WOULD MAKE TODAY GREAT?

1. _____
2. _____
3. _____

MINDFULNESS

HOW DO I FEEL TODAY? _____

_____

_____

_____

MY MOOD IS...

- ☐ HAPPY
- ☐ FOCUSED
- ☐ ENERGETIC
- ☐ EXCITED
- ☐ SAD
- ☐ TIRED
- ☐ ANXIOUS
- ☐ ANGRY

I PRACTICED...

- ☐ MEDITATION
- ☐ LOVING SELF-TALK
- ☐ DEEP BREATHING

FITNESS

EXERCISE _____

_____

_____

_____

RATE MY...

- ENERGY LEVEL ★ ★ ★
- SELF-CARE ★ ★ ★
- HUNGER/CRAVINGS ★ ★ ★
- RELATIONSHIP WITH FOOD & EXERCISE ★ ★ ★

ONE THING I WOULD LIKE TO KEEP WORKING ON _____

_____

_____

3 THINGS I AM GRATEFUL FOR TODAY

1. _____
2. _____
3. _____

☐ RECORD BODY MEASUREMENTS | # OF STEPS | % BODY FAT | WEIGHT

Tuesday
WEEK 1

___/___/___

NUTRITION

		PROTEIN	STARCH	FRUIT	VEGETABLES	FATS
BREAKFAST 🕐						
MORNING SNACK 🕐						
LUNCH 🕐						
AFTERNOON SNACK 🕐						
DINNER 🕐						
EVENING SNACK 🕐						
TOTALS						

WATER 💧 2 3 4 5 6 7 8 ➕ ➕ ➕ ➕

OTHER BEVERAGES _____

SUPPLEMENTS/MEDICATIONS _____

DIGESTION/BOWEL MOVEMENTS _____

*"GO CONFIDENTLY IN THE DIRECTION OF YOUR DREAMS!
LIVE THE LIFE YOU'VE IMAGINED."
- HENRY DAVID THOREAU*

WHAT WOULD MAKE TODAY GREAT?

1. _____
2. _____
3. _____

MINDFULNESS

HOW DO I FEEL TODAY? _____
_____
_____
_____

MY MOOD IS...

- ☐ HAPPY
- ☐ FOCUSED
- ☐ ENERGETIC
- ☐ EXCITED
- ☐ SAD
- ☐ TIRED
- ☐ ANXIOUS
- ☐ ANGRY

I PRACTICED...

- ☐ MEDITATION
- ☐ LOVING SELF-TALK
- ☐ DEEP BREATHING

FITNESS

EXERCISE _____
_____
_____
_____

RATE MY...

- ENERGY LEVEL ☆☆☆
- SELF-CARE ☆☆☆
- HUNGER/CRAVINGS ☆☆☆
- RELATIONSHIP WITH FOOD & EXERCISE ☆☆☆

ONE THING I WOULD LIKE TO KEEP WORKING ON _____
_____
_____

3 THINGS I AM GRATEFUL FOR TODAY

1. _____
2. _____
3. _____

| # OF STEPS | | % BODY FAT | | WEIGHT | |

Wednesday ___/___/___
WEEK 1

NUTRITION

		PROTEIN	STARCH	FRUIT	VEGETABLES	FATS
BREAKFAST 🕐						
MORNING SNACK 🕐						
LUNCH 🕐						
AFTERNOON SNACK 🕐						
DINNER 🕐						
EVENING SNACK 🕐						
TOTALS						

WATER 🍊 ② ③ ④ ⑤ ⑥ ⑦ ⑧ ⊕ ⊕ ⊕ ⊕

OTHER BEVERAGES _____

SUPPLEMENTS/MEDICATIONS _____

DIGESTION/BOWEL MOVEMENTS _____

> "LEAVE THE IRREPARABLE PAST BEHIND, AND STEP FORTH INTO THE INVINCIBLE FUTURE."
> - OSWALD CHAMBERS

WHAT WOULD MAKE TODAY GREAT?

1. _____
2. _____
3. _____

MINDFULNESS

HOW DO I FEEL TODAY? _____
_____
_____
_____

MY MOOD IS...

- ☐ HAPPY
- ☐ FOCUSED
- ☐ ENERGETIC
- ☐ EXCITED
- ☐ SAD
- ☐ TIRED
- ☐ ANXIOUS
- ☐ ANGRY

FITNESS

EXERCISE _____
_____
_____
_____

I PRACTICED...

- ☐ MEDITATION
- ☐ LOVING SELF-TALK
- ☐ DEEP BREATHING

RATE MY...

- ENERGY LEVEL ☆☆☆
- SELF-CARE ☆☆☆
- HUNGER/CRAVINGS ☆☆☆
- RELATIONSHIP WITH FOOD & EXERCISE ☆☆☆

ONE THING I WOULD LIKE TO KEEP WORKING ON _____
_____
_____

3 THINGS I AM GRATEFUL FOR TODAY

1. _____
2. _____
3. _____

# OF STEPS	% BODY FAT	WEIGHT

Thursday

WEEK 1

___/___/___

NUTRITION

		PROTEIN	STARCH	FRUIT	VEGETABLES	FATS
BREAKFAST 🕐						
MORNING SNACK 🕐						
LUNCH 🕐						
AFTERNOON SNACK 🕐						
DINNER 🕐						
EVENING SNACK 🕐						
TOTALS						

WATER 🍋 2 3 4 5 6 7 8 ⊕ ⊕ ⊕ ⊕

OTHER BEVERAGES _____

SUPPLEMENTS/MEDICATIONS _____

DIGESTION/BOWEL MOVEMENTS _____

> "THE SECRET OF GETTING AHEAD IS
> GETTING STARTED."
> - MARK TWAIN

WHAT WOULD MAKE TODAY GREAT?

1. _____
2. _____
3. _____

MINDFULNESS

HOW DO I FEEL TODAY? _____
_____
_____
_____

MY MOOD IS...

- ☐ HAPPY
- ☐ FOCUSED
- ☐ ENERGETIC
- ☐ EXCITED
- ☐ SAD
- ☐ TIRED
- ☐ ANXIOUS
- ☐ ANGRY

I PRACTICED...

- ☐ MEDITATION
- ☐ LOVING SELF-TALK
- ☐ DEEP BREATHING

FITNESS

EXERCISE _____
_____
_____
_____

RATE MY...

- ENERGY LEVEL ☆ ☆ ☆
- SELF-CARE ☆ ☆ ☆
- HUNGER/CRAVINGS ☆ ☆ ☆
- RELATIONSHIP WITH FOOD & EXERCISE ☆ ☆ ☆

ONE THING I WOULD LIKE TO KEEP WORKING ON _____
_____
_____

3 THINGS I AM GRATEFUL FOR TODAY

1. _____
2. _____
3. _____

# OF STEPS		% BODY FAT		WEIGHT	

Friday
WEEK 1

___/___/___

NUTRITION

	PROTEIN	STARCH	FRUIT	VEGETABLES	FATS
BREAKFAST 🕐					
MORNING SNACK 🕐					
LUNCH 🕐					
AFTERNOON SNACK 🕐					
DINNER 🕐					
EVENING SNACK 🕐					
TOTALS					

WATER 🍊 ② ③ ④ ⑤ ⑥ ⑦ ⑧ ⊕ ⊕ ⊕ ⊕

OTHER BEVERAGES _____

SUPPLEMENTS/MEDICATIONS _____

DIGESTION/BOWEL MOVEMENTS _____

> "THE BEST TIME TO PLANT A TREE WAS 20 YEARS AGO.
> THE SECOND BEST TIME IS NOW."
> - CHINESE PROVERB

WHAT WOULD MAKE TODAY GREAT?

1. _____
2. _____
3. _____

MINDFULNESS

HOW DO I FEEL TODAY? _____
_____
_____
_____

MY MOOD IS...

☐ HAPPY   ☐ SAD
☐ FOCUSED   ☐ TIRED
☐ ENERGETIC ☐ ANXIOUS
☐ EXCITED   ☐ ANGRY

FITNESS

EXERCISE _____
_____
_____
_____

I PRACTICED...

☐ MEDITATION
☐ LOVING SELF-TALK
☐ DEEP BREATHING

RATE MY...

ENERGY LEVEL ★ ★ ★
SELF-CARE ★ ★ ★
HUNGER/CRAVINGS ★ ★ ★
RELATIONSHIP WITH FOOD & EXERCISE ★ ★ ★

ONE THING I WOULD LIKE TO KEEP WORKING ON _____
_____
_____

3 THINGS I AM GRATEFUL FOR TODAY

1. _____
2. _____
3. _____

# OF STEPS		% BODY FAT		WEIGHT	

saturday
WEEK 1   ___/___/___

NUTRITION

		PROTEIN	STARCH	FRUIT	VEGETABLES	FATS
BREAKFAST 🕐						
MORNING SNACK 🕐						
LUNCH 🕐						
AFTERNOON SNACK 🕐						
DINNER 🕐						
EVENING SNACK 🕐						
TOTALS						

WATER 🍊 ② ③ ④ ⑤ ⑥ ⑦ ⑧ ⊕ ⊕ ⊕ ⊕

OTHER BEVERAGES _____

SUPPLEMENTS/MEDICATIONS _____

DIGESTION/BOWEL MOVEMENTS _____

> "ENERGY AND PERSISTENCE CONQUER ALL THINGS."
> - BENJAMIN FRANKLIN

WHAT WOULD MAKE TODAY GREAT?

1. _____
2. _____
3. _____

FITNESS

EXERCISE _____

_____

_____

_____

RATE MY...

- ENERGY LEVEL ☆☆☆
- SELF-CARE ☆☆☆
- HUNGER/CRAVINGS ☆☆☆
- RELATIONSHIP WITH FOOD & EXERCISE ☆☆☆

ONE THING I WOULD LIKE TO KEEP WORKING ON _____

_____

MINDFULNESS

HOW DO I FEEL TODAY? _____

_____

_____

_____

MY MOOD IS...

- ☐ HAPPY
- ☐ FOCUSED
- ☐ ENERGETIC
- ☐ EXCITED
- ☐ SAD
- ☐ TIRED
- ☐ ANXIOUS
- ☐ ANGRY

I PRACTICED...

- ☐ MEDITATION
- ☐ LOVING SELF-TALK
- ☐ DEEP BREATHING

3 THINGS I AM GRATEFUL FOR TODAY

1. _____
2. _____
3. _____

# OF STEPS	% BODY FAT	WEIGHT

Sunday
WEEK 1

___/___/___

NUTRITION

	PROTEIN	STARCH	FRUIT	VEGETABLES	FATS
BREAKFAST					
MORNING SNACK					
LUNCH					
AFTERNOON SNACK					
DINNER					
EVENING SNACK					
TOTALS					

WATER ◯ 2 3 4 5 6 7 8 ⊕ ⊕ ⊕ ⊕

OTHER BEVERAGES _____

SUPPLEMENTS/MEDICATIONS _____

DIGESTION/BOWEL MOVEMENTS _____

**ASK YOURSELF TODAY:
WHAT AM I PROUD OF MYSELF FOR ACCOMPLISHING
THIS PAST WEEK?**

WHAT WOULD MAKE TODAY GREAT?

1) _____
2) _____
3) _____

MINDFULNESS

HOW DO I FEEL TODAY? _____
_____
_____
_____

MY MOOD IS...

- ☐ HAPPY
- ☐ FOCUSED
- ☐ ENERGETIC
- ☐ EXCITED
- ☐ SAD
- ☐ TIRED
- ☐ ANXIOUS
- ☐ ANGRY

FITNESS

EXERCISE _____
_____
_____
_____

I PRACTICED...

- ☐ MEDITATION
- ☐ LOVING SELF-TALK
- ☐ DEEP BREATHING

RATE MY...

- ENERGY LEVEL ☆ ☆ ☆
- SELF-CARE ☆ ☆ ☆
- HUNGER/CRAVINGS ☆ ☆ ☆
- RELATIONSHIP WITH FOOD & EXERCISE ☆ ☆ ☆

ONE THING I WOULD LIKE TO KEEP WORKING ON _____
_____
_____

3 THINGS I AM GRATEFUL FOR TODAY

1) _____
2) _____
3) _____

| # OF STEPS | | % BODY FAT | | WEIGHT | |

I AM...
WORTHY

*"YOUR GREATEST DREAMS ARE ALL ON THE OTHER SIDE
OF THE WALL OF FEAR AND CAUTION."
- UNKNOWN*

WHAT WOULD MAKE TODAY GREAT?

1. _____
2. _____
3. _____

MINDFULNESS

HOW DO I FEEL TODAY? _____
_____
_____
_____

MY MOOD IS...

☐ HAPPY ☐ SAD
☐ FOCUSED ☐ TIRED
☐ ENERGETIC ☐ ANXIOUS
☐ EXCITED ☐ ANGRY

I PRACTICED...

☐ MEDITATION
☐ LOVING SELF-TALK
☐ DEEP BREATHING

FITNESS

EXERCISE _____
_____
_____
_____

RATE MY...

ENERGY LEVEL ☆ ☆ ☆
SELF-CARE ☆ ☆ ☆
HUNGER/CRAVINGS ☆ ☆ ☆
RELATIONSHIP WITH
FOOD & EXERCISE ☆ ☆ ☆

ONE THING I WOULD LIKE TO KEEP WORKING ON _____
_____
_____

3 THINGS I AM GRATEFUL FOR TODAY

1. _____
2. _____
3. _____

| # OF STEPS | | % BODY FAT | | WEIGHT | |

Tuesday
WEEK 2

___/___/___

NUTRITION

	PROTEIN	STARCH	FRUIT	VEGETABLES	FATS
BREAKFAST 🕐					
MORNING SNACK 🕐					
LUNCH 🕐					
AFTERNOON SNACK 🕐					
DINNER 🕐					
EVENING SNACK 🕐					
TOTALS					

WATER 💧 ② ③ ④ ⑤ ⑥ ⑦ ⑧ ⊕ ⊕ ⊕ ⊕

OTHER BEVERAGES _____

SUPPLEMENTS/MEDICATIONS _____

DIGESTION/BOWEL MOVEMENTS _____

*"TO KEEP THE BODY IN GOOD HEALTH IS A DUTY...
OTHERWISE WE SHALL NOT BE ABLE TO KEEP OUR
MIND STRONG AND CLEAR."
- GAUTAMA BUDDHA*

WHAT WOULD MAKE TODAY GREAT?

1. _____
2. _____
3. _____

MINDFULNESS

HOW DO I FEEL TODAY? _____
_____
_____
_____

MY MOOD IS...

- ☐ HAPPY
- ☐ FOCUSED
- ☐ ENERGETIC
- ☐ EXCITED
- ☐ SAD
- ☐ TIRED
- ☐ ANXIOUS
- ☐ ANGRY

I PRACTICED...

- ☐ MEDITATION
- ☐ LOVING SELF-TALK
- ☐ DEEP BREATHING

FITNESS

EXERCISE _____
_____
_____
_____

RATE MY...

- ENERGY LEVEL ☆☆☆
- SELF-CARE ☆☆☆
- HUNGER/CRAVINGS ☆☆☆
- RELATIONSHIP WITH FOOD & EXERCISE ☆☆☆

ONE THING I WOULD LIKE TO KEEP WORKING ON _____
_____
_____

3 THINGS I AM GRATEFUL FOR TODAY

1. _____
2. _____
3. _____

# OF STEPS		% BODY FAT		WEIGHT	

Wednesday ___/___/___
WEEK 2

NUTRITION

		PROTEIN	STARCH	FRUIT	VEGETABLES	FATS
BREAKFAST 🕐						
MORNING SNACK 🕐						
LUNCH 🕐						
AFTERNOON SNACK 🕐						
DINNER 🕐						
EVENING SNACK 🕐						
TOTALS						

WATER 💧 ② ③ ④ ⑤ ⑥ ⑦ ⑧ ⊕ ⊕ ⊕ ⊕

OTHER BEVERAGES _____

SUPPLEMENTS/MEDICATIONS _____

DIGESTION/BOWEL MOVEMENTS _____

"KEEP MOVING FORWARD, ONE STEP AT A TIME."
- UNKNOWN

WHAT WOULD MAKE TODAY GREAT?

1. _____
2. _____
3. _____

MINDFULNESS

HOW DO I FEEL TODAY? _____
_____
_____
_____

MY MOOD IS...

- ☐ HAPPY
- ☐ FOCUSED
- ☐ ENERGETIC
- ☐ EXCITED
- ☐ SAD
- ☐ TIRED
- ☐ ANXIOUS
- ☐ ANGRY

I PRACTICED...

- ☐ MEDITATION
- ☐ LOVING SELF-TALK
- ☐ DEEP BREATHING

FITNESS

EXERCISE _____
_____
_____
_____

RATE MY...

- ENERGY LEVEL ☆☆☆
- SELF-CARE ☆☆☆
- HUNGER/CRAVINGS ☆☆☆
- RELATIONSHIP WITH FOOD & EXERCISE ☆☆☆

ONE THING I WOULD LIKE TO KEEP WORKING ON _____
_____
_____

3 THINGS I AM GRATEFUL FOR TODAY

1. _____
2. _____
3. _____

# OF STEPS	% BODY FAT	WEIGHT

Thursday
WEEK 2

___/___/___

NUTRITION

	PROTEIN	STARCH	FRUIT	VEGETABLES	FATS
BREAKFAST 🕐					
MORNING SNACK 🕐					
LUNCH 🕐					
AFTERNOON SNACK 🕐					
DINNER 🕐					
EVENING SNACK 🕐					
TOTALS					

WATER ① ② ③ ④ ⑤ ⑥ ⑦ ⑧ ⊕ ⊕ ⊕ ⊕

OTHER BEVERAGES _____

SUPPLEMENTS/MEDICATIONS _____

DIGESTION/BOWEL MOVEMENTS _____

"LEARNING IS NOT ATTAINED BY CHANCE, IT MUST BE SOUGHT FOR WITH ARDOR AND DILIGENCE."
- ABIGAIL ADAMS

WHAT WOULD MAKE TODAY GREAT?

1. _____
2. _____
3. _____

FITNESS

EXERCISE _____
_____
_____
_____

RATE MY...

- ENERGY LEVEL ☆☆☆
- SELF-CARE ☆☆☆
- HUNGER/CRAVINGS ☆☆☆
- RELATIONSHIP WITH FOOD & EXERCISE ☆☆☆

ONE THING I WOULD LIKE TO KEEP WORKING ON _____
_____
_____

MINDFULNESS

HOW DO I FEEL TODAY? _____
_____
_____
_____

MY MOOD IS...

- ☐ HAPPY   ☐ SAD
- ☐ FOCUSED   ☐ TIRED
- ☐ ENERGETIC   ☐ ANXIOUS
- ☐ EXCITED   ☐ ANGRY

I PRACTICED...

- ☐ MEDITATION
- ☐ LOVING SELF-TALK
- ☐ DEEP BREATHING

3 THINGS I AM GRATEFUL FOR TODAY

1. _____
2. _____
3. _____

# OF STEPS	% BODY FAT	WEIGHT

Friday
WEEK 2

___/___/___

NUTRITION

	PROTEIN	STARCH	FRUIT	VEGETABLES	FATS
BREAKFAST 🕐					
MORNING SNACK 🕐					
LUNCH 🕐					
AFTERNOON SNACK 🕐					
DINNER 🕐					
EVENING SNACK 🕐					
TOTALS					

WATER 🍋 2 3 4 5 6 7 8 ➕ ➕ ➕ ➕

OTHER BEVERAGES _____

SUPPLEMENTS/MEDICATIONS _____

DIGESTION/BOWEL MOVEMENTS _____

> "ANYONE WHO HAS A WHY TO LIVE CAN BEAR ALMOST ANY WHAT."
> - NIETZCHE

WHAT WOULD MAKE TODAY GREAT?

1. _____
2. _____
3. _____

MINDFULNESS

HOW DO I FEEL TODAY? _____
_____
_____
_____

MY MOOD IS...

- ☐ HAPPY
- ☐ FOCUSED
- ☐ ENERGETIC
- ☐ EXCITED
- ☐ SAD
- ☐ TIRED
- ☐ ANXIOUS
- ☐ ANGRY

FITNESS

EXERCISE _____
_____
_____
_____

I PRACTICED...

- ☐ MEDITATION
- ☐ LOVING SELF-TALK
- ☐ DEEP BREATHING

RATE MY...

- ENERGY LEVEL ☆☆☆
- SELF-CARE ☆☆☆
- HUNGER/CRAVINGS ☆☆☆
- RELATIONSHIP WITH FOOD & EXERCISE ☆☆☆

ONE THING I WOULD LIKE TO KEEP WORKING ON _____
_____
_____

3 THINGS I AM GRATEFUL FOR TODAY

1. _____
2. _____
3. _____

☐ RECORD BODY MEASUREMENTS | # OF STEPS ____ | % BODY FAT ____ | WEIGHT ____

saturday ___/___/___
WEEK 2

NUTRITION

	PROTEIN	STARCH	FRUIT	VEGETABLES	FATS
BREAKFAST 🕐					
MORNING SNACK 🕐					
LUNCH 🕐					
AFTERNOON SNACK 🕐					
DINNER 🕐					
EVENING SNACK 🕐					
TOTALS					

WATER 🍋 ② ③ ④ ⑤ ⑥ ⑦ ⑧ ⊕ ⊕ ⊕ ⊕

OTHER BEVERAGES _____

SUPPLEMENTS/MEDICATIONS _____

DIGESTION/BOWEL MOVEMENTS _____

"AND SUDDENLY YOU KNOW: IT'S TIME TO START SOMETHING NEW AND TRUST THE MAGIC OF BEGINNINGS."
- MEISTER ECKHART

WHAT WOULD MAKE TODAY GREAT?

1. _____
2. _____
3. _____

MINDFULNESS

HOW DO I FEEL TODAY? _____
_____
_____
_____

MY MOOD IS...

- ☐ HAPPY
- ☐ FOCUSED
- ☐ ENERGETIC
- ☐ EXCITED
- ☐ SAD
- ☐ TIRED
- ☐ ANXIOUS
- ☐ ANGRY

FITNESS

EXERCISE _____
_____
_____
_____

I PRACTICED...

- ☐ MEDITATION
- ☐ LOVING SELF-TALK
- ☐ DEEP BREATHING

RATE MY...

ENERGY LEVEL	☆ ☆ ☆	
SELF-CARE	☆ ☆ ☆	
HUNGER/CRAVINGS	☆ ☆ ☆	
RELATIONSHIP WITH FOOD & EXERCISE	☆ ☆ ☆	

ONE THING I WOULD LIKE TO KEEP WORKING ON _____
_____
_____

3 THINGS I AM GRATEFUL FOR TODAY

1. _____
2. _____
3. _____

# OF STEPS		% BODY FAT		WEIGHT	

Sunday
WEEK 2

___/___/___

NUTRITION

	PROTEIN	STARCH	FRUIT	VEGETABLES	FATS
BREAKFAST 🕐					
MORNING SNACK 🕐					
LUNCH 🕐					
AFTERNOON SNACK 🕐					
DINNER 🕐					
EVENING SNACK 🕐					
TOTALS					

WATER 💧 ② ③ ④ ⑤ ⑥ ⑦ ⑧ ➕ ➕ ➕

OTHER BEVERAGES _____

SUPPLEMENTS/MEDICATIONS _____

DIGESTION/BOWEL MOVEMENTS _____

**ASK YOURSELF TODAY:
WHAT CAN I DO TODAY TO MAKE MY WEEK
FLOW WITH EASE?**

WHAT WOULD MAKE TODAY GREAT?

1. _____
2. _____
3. _____

MINDFULNESS

HOW DO I FEEL TODAY? _____
_____
_____
_____

MY MOOD IS...
- ☐ HAPPY
- ☐ FOCUSED
- ☐ ENERGETIC
- ☐ EXCITED
- ☐ SAD
- ☐ TIRED
- ☐ ANXIOUS
- ☐ ANGRY

I PRACTICED...
- ☐ MEDITATION
- ☐ LOVING SELF-TALK
- ☐ DEEP BREATHING

FITNESS

EXERCISE _____
_____
_____
_____

RATE MY...

ENERGY LEVEL	☆	☆	☆
SELF-CARE	☆	☆	☆
HUNGER/CRAVINGS	☆	☆	☆
RELATIONSHIP WITH FOOD & EXERCISE	☆	☆	☆

ONE THING I WOULD LIKE TO KEEP WORKING ON _____
_____
_____

3 THINGS I AM GRATEFUL FOR TODAY

1. _____
2. _____
3. _____

# OF STEPS		% BODY FAT		WEIGHT	

I AM...
CAPABLE

Week 3

Week 3 GOALS

GOALS FOR THIS WEEK

1. _____
2. _____
3. _____

EXERCISE PLAN

Day	
MONDAY	_____
TUESDAY	_____
WEDNESDAY	_____
THURSDAY	_____
FRIDAY	_____
SATURDAY	_____
SUNDAY	_____

Week 3
MEAL PLAN & GROCERY LIST

MONDAY
- B
- L
- D
- SNACKS

TUESDAY
- B
- L
- D
- SNACKS

WEDNESDAY
- B
- L
- D
- SNACKS

THURSDAY
- B
- L
- D
- SNACKS

FRIDAY
- B
- L
- D
- SNACKS

SATURDAY
- B
- L
- D
- SNACKS

SUNDAY
- B
- L
- D
- SNACKS

GROCERY LIST

Monday
WEEK 3

___/___/___

NUTRITION

	PROTEIN	STARCH	FRUIT	VEGETABLES	FATS
BREAKFAST 🕐					
MORNING SNACK 🕐					
LUNCH 🕐					
AFTERNOON SNACK 🕐					
DINNER 🕐					
EVENING SNACK 🕐					
TOTALS					

WATER 🍊 ② ③ ④ ⑤ ⑥ ⑦ ⑧ ⊕ ⊕ ⊕ ⊕

OTHER BEVERAGES _____

SUPPLEMENTS/MEDICATIONS _____

DIGESTION/BOWEL MOVEMENTS _____

"IT'S NOT THE STRAINING FOR GREAT THINGS THAT IS MOST EFFECTIVE; IT IS THE DOING THE LITTLE THINGS, THE COMMON DUTIES, A LITTLE BETTER AND BETTER."
- ELIZABETH STUART PHELPS

WHAT WOULD MAKE TODAY GREAT?

1. _____
2. _____
3. _____

MINDFULNESS

HOW DO I FEEL TODAY? _____
_____
_____
_____

MY MOOD IS...
- ☐ HAPPY
- ☐ FOCUSED
- ☐ ENERGETIC
- ☐ EXCITED
- ☐ SAD
- ☐ TIRED
- ☐ ANXIOUS
- ☐ ANGRY

I PRACTICED...
- ☐ MEDITATION
- ☐ LOVING SELF-TALK
- ☐ DEEP BREATHING

FITNESS

EXERCISE _____
_____
_____

RATE MY...

ENERGY LEVEL	☆ ☆ ☆
SELF-CARE	☆ ☆ ☆
HUNGER/CRAVINGS	☆ ☆ ☆
RELATIONSHIP WITH FOOD & EXERCISE	☆ ☆ ☆

ONE THING I WOULD LIKE TO KEEP WORKING ON _____
_____
_____

3 THINGS I AM GRATEFUL FOR TODAY

1. _____
2. _____
3. _____

# OF STEPS	% BODY FAT	WEIGHT

Tuesday
WEEK 3

___/___/___

NUTRITION

	PROTEIN	STARCH	FRUIT	VEGETABLES	FATS
BREAKFAST 🕐					
MORNING SNACK 🕐					
LUNCH 🕐					
AFTERNOON SNACK 🕐					
DINNER 🕐					
EVENING SNACK 🕐					
TOTALS					

WATER ① ② ③ ④ ⑤ ⑥ ⑦ ⑧ ⊕ ⊕ ⊕ ⊕

OTHER BEVERAGES _____

SUPPLEMENTS/MEDICATIONS _____

DIGESTION/BOWEL MOVEMENTS _____

> "THOSE WHO THINK THEY CAN AND THOSE WHO THINK THEY CAN'T ARE BOTH USUALLY RIGHT."
> - CONFUCIOUS

WHAT WOULD MAKE TODAY GREAT?

1. _____
2. _____
3. _____

MINDFULNESS

HOW DO I FEEL TODAY? _____

_____
_____
_____

MY MOOD IS...

- ☐ HAPPY
- ☐ FOCUSED
- ☐ ENERGETIC
- ☐ EXCITED
- ☐ SAD
- ☐ TIRED
- ☐ ANXIOUS
- ☐ ANGRY

FITNESS

EXERCISE _____
_____
_____
_____

I PRACTICED...

- ☐ MEDITATION
- ☐ LOVING SELF-TALK
- ☐ DEEP BREATHING

RATE MY...

ENERGY LEVEL	☆ ☆ ☆
SELF-CARE	☆ ☆ ☆
HUNGER/CRAVINGS	☆ ☆ ☆
RELATIONSHIP WITH FOOD & EXERCISE	☆ ☆ ☆

ONE THING I WOULD LIKE TO KEEP WORKING ON _____
_____
_____

3 THINGS I AM GRATEFUL FOR TODAY

1. _____
2. _____
3. _____

# OF STEPS		% BODY FAT		WEIGHT	

Wednesday ___/___/___
WEEK 3

NUTRITION

		PROTEIN	STARCH	FRUIT	VEGETABLES	FATS
BREAKFAST 🕐						
MORNING SNACK 🕐						
LUNCH 🕐						
AFTERNOON SNACK 🕐						
DINNER 🕐						
EVENING SNACK 🕐						
TOTALS						

WATER 🍊 ② ③ ④ ⑤ ⑥ ⑦ ⑧ ⊕ ⊕ ⊕

OTHER BEVERAGES _____

SUPPLEMENTS/MEDICATIONS _____

DIGESTION/BOWEL MOVEMENTS _____

"DO MORE WITH LESS."
- UNKNOWN

WHAT WOULD MAKE TODAY GREAT?

1. _____
2. _____
3. _____

MINDFULNESS

HOW DO I FEEL TODAY? _____
_____
_____
_____

MY MOOD IS...

- ☐ HAPPY
- ☐ FOCUSED
- ☐ ENERGETIC
- ☐ EXCITED
- ☐ SAD
- ☐ TIRED
- ☐ ANXIOUS
- ☐ ANGRY

FITNESS

EXERCISE _____
_____
_____
_____

I PRACTICED...

- ☐ MEDITATION
- ☐ LOVING SELF-TALK
- ☐ DEEP BREATHING

RATE MY...

- ENERGY LEVEL ☆☆☆
- SELF-CARE ☆☆☆
- HUNGER/CRAVINGS ☆☆☆
- RELATIONSHIP WITH FOOD & EXERCISE ☆☆☆

ONE THING I WOULD LIKE TO KEEP WORKING ON _____
_____
_____

3 THINGS I AM GRATEFUL FOR TODAY

1. _____
2. _____
3. _____

# OF STEPS	% BODY FAT	WEIGHT

Thursday ___/___/___
WEEK 3

NUTRITION

		PROTEIN	STARCH	FRUIT	VEGETABLES	FATS
BREAKFAST 🕐						
MORNING SNACK 🕐						
LUNCH 🕐						
AFTERNOON SNACK 🕐						
DINNER 🕐						
EVENING SNACK 🕐						
TOTALS						

WATER 💧 2 3 4 5 6 7 8 ➕ ➕ ➕ ➕

OTHER BEVERAGES _____

SUPPLEMENTS/MEDICATIONS _____

DIGESTION/BOWEL MOVEMENTS _____

> "SIMPLICITY IS THE ULTIMATE SOPHISTICATION."
> - LEONARDO DA VINCI

MINDFULNESS

HOW DO I FEEL TODAY? _____

_____

_____

_____

MY MOOD IS...

- ☐ HAPPY
- ☐ FOCUSED
- ☐ ENERGETIC
- ☐ EXCITED
- ☐ SAD
- ☐ TIRED
- ☐ ANXIOUS
- ☐ ANGRY

I PRACTICED...

- ☐ MEDITATION
- ☐ LOVING SELF-TALK
- ☐ DEEP BREATHING

WHAT WOULD MAKE TODAY GREAT?

1. _____
2. _____
3. _____

FITNESS

EXERCISE _____

_____

_____

_____

RATE MY...

- ENERGY LEVEL ☆ ☆ ☆
- SELF-CARE ☆ ☆ ☆
- HUNGER/CRAVINGS ☆ ☆ ☆
- RELATIONSHIP WITH FOOD & EXERCISE ☆ ☆ ☆

ONE THING I WOULD LIKE TO KEEP WORKING ON _____

_____

_____

3 THINGS I AM GRATEFUL FOR TODAY

1. _____
2. _____
3. _____

# OF STEPS		% BODY FAT		WEIGHT	

Friday
WEEK 3

___/___/___

NUTRITION

		PROTEIN	STARCH	FRUIT	VEGETABLES	FATS
BREAKFAST 🕐						
MORNING SNACK 🕐						
LUNCH 🕐						
AFTERNOON SNACK 🕐						
DINNER 🕐						
EVENING SNACK 🕐						
TOTALS						

WATER 🍊 ② ③ ④ ⑤ ⑥ ⑦ ⑧ ⊕ ⊕ ⊕ ⊕

OTHER BEVERAGES _____

SUPPLEMENTS/MEDICATIONS _____

DIGESTION/BOWEL MOVEMENTS _____

*"DON'T JUDGE EACH DAY BY THE HARVEST
THAT YOU REAP BUT BY THE SEEDS THAT YOU PLANT."
- ROBERT LOUIS STEVENSON*

WHAT WOULD MAKE TODAY GREAT?

1. _____
2. _____
3. _____

MINDFULNESS

HOW DO I FEEL TODAY? _____
_____
_____
_____

MY MOOD IS...

- ☐ HAPPY   ☐ SAD
- ☐ FOCUSED   ☐ TIRED
- ☐ ENERGETIC   ☐ ANXIOUS
- ☐ EXCITED   ☐ ANGRY

I PRACTICED...

- ☐ MEDITATION
- ☐ LOVING SELF-TALK
- ☐ DEEP BREATHING

FITNESS

EXERCISE _____
_____
_____
_____

RATE MY...

- ENERGY LEVEL ☆ ☆ ☆
- SELF-CARE ☆ ☆ ☆
- HUNGER/CRAVINGS ☆ ☆ ☆
- RELATIONSHIP WITH FOOD & EXERCISE ☆ ☆ ☆

ONE THING I WOULD LIKE TO KEEP WORKING ON _____
_____
_____

3 THINGS I AM GRATEFUL FOR TODAY

1. _____
2. _____
3. _____

# OF STEPS	% BODY FAT	WEIGHT

saturday
WEEK 3

___/___/___

NUTRITION

		PROTEIN	STARCH	FRUIT	VEGETABLES	FATS
BREAKFAST 🕐						
MORNING SNACK 🕐						
LUNCH 🕐						
AFTERNOON SNACK 🕐						
DINNER 🕐						
EVENING SNACK 🕐						
TOTALS						

WATER 🍊 ② ③ ④ ⑤ ⑥ ⑦ ⑧ ⊕ ⊕ ⊕ ⊕

OTHER BEVERAGES _____

SUPPLEMENTS/MEDICATIONS _____

DIGESTION/BOWEL MOVEMENTS _____

> "I'M NOT AFRAID OF STORMS,
> FOR I'M LEARNING HOW TO SAIL MY SHIP."
> - LOUISA MAY ALCOTT

WHAT WOULD MAKE TODAY GREAT?

1. _____
2. _____
3. _____

MINDFULNESS

HOW DO I FEEL TODAY? _____

_____

_____

_____

MY MOOD IS...

- ☐ HAPPY
- ☐ FOCUSED
- ☐ ENERGETIC
- ☐ EXCITED
- ☐ SAD
- ☐ TIRED
- ☐ ANXIOUS
- ☐ ANGRY

I PRACTICED...

- ☐ MEDITATION
- ☐ LOVING SELF-TALK
- ☐ DEEP BREATHING

FITNESS

EXERCISE _____

_____

_____

_____

RATE MY...

- ENERGY LEVEL ☆ ☆ ☆
- SELF-CARE ☆ ☆ ☆
- HUNGER/CRAVINGS ☆ ☆ ☆
- RELATIONSHIP WITH FOOD & EXERCISE ☆ ☆ ☆

ONE THING I WOULD LIKE TO KEEP WORKING ON _____

_____

_____

3 THINGS I AM GRATEFUL FOR TODAY

1. _____
2. _____
3. _____

# OF STEPS		% BODY FAT		WEIGHT	

Sunday
WEEK 3

___/___/___

NUTRITION

		PROTEIN	STARCH	FRUIT	VEGETABLES	FATS
BREAKFAST 🕐						
MORNING SNACK 🕐						
LUNCH 🕐						
AFTERNOON SNACK 🕐						
DINNER 🕐						
EVENING SNACK 🕐						
TOTALS						

WATER 🍊 ② ③ ④ ⑤ ⑥ ⑦ ⑧ ⊕ ⊕ ⊕ ⊕

OTHER BEVERAGES _____

SUPPLEMENTS/MEDICATIONS _____

DIGESTION/BOWEL MOVEMENTS _____

ASK YOURSELF TODAY:
WHEN DID I FEEL MOST ALIGNED WITH MY GOALS THIS PAST WEEK?

WHAT WOULD MAKE TODAY GREAT?

1. _____
2. _____
3. _____

MINDFULNESS

HOW DO I FEEL TODAY? _____

_____
_____
_____

MY MOOD IS...

- ☐ HAPPY
- ☐ FOCUSED
- ☐ ENERGETIC
- ☐ EXCITED
- ☐ SAD
- ☐ TIRED
- ☐ ANXIOUS
- ☐ ANGRY

I PRACTICED...

- ☐ MEDITATION
- ☐ LOVING SELF-TALK
- ☐ DEEP BREATHING

FITNESS

EXERCISE _____

_____
_____
_____

RATE MY...

- ENERGY LEVEL ☆☆☆
- SELF-CARE ☆☆☆
- HUNGER/CRAVINGS ☆☆☆
- RELATIONSHIP WITH FOOD & EXERCISE ☆☆☆

ONE THING I WOULD LIKE TO KEEP WORKING ON _____

_____
_____

3 THINGS I AM GRATEFUL FOR TODAY

1. _____
2. _____
3. _____

# OF STEPS	% BODY FAT	WEIGHT

I AM...

MINDFUL

Week 4

Week 4 GOALS

GOALS FOR THIS WEEK

1. _____
2. _____
3. _____

EXERCISE PLAN

MONDAY	_____
TUESDAY	_____
WEDNESDAY	_____
THURSDAY	_____
FRIDAY	_____
SATURDAY	_____
SUNDAY	_____

Week 4
MEAL PLAN & GROCERY LIST

MONDAY
- (B)
- (L)
- (D)
- SNACKS

TUESDAY
- (B)
- (L)
- (D)
- SNACKS

WEDNESDAY
- (B)
- (L)
- (D)
- SNACKS

THURSDAY
- (B)
- (L)
- (D)
- SNACKS

FRIDAY
- (B)
- (L)
- (D)
- SNACKS

SATURDAY
- (B)
- (L)
- (D)
- SNACKS

SUNDAY
- (B)
- (L)
- (D)
- SNACKS

GROCERY LIST

Monday
WEEK 4

___/___/___

NUTRITION

	PROTEIN	STARCH	FRUIT	VEGETABLES	FATS
BREAKFAST 🕐					
MORNING SNACK 🕐					
LUNCH 🕐					
AFTERNOON SNACK 🕐					
DINNER 🕐					
EVENING SNACK 🕐					
TOTALS					

WATER ⊛ ② ③ ④ ⑤ ⑥ ⑦ ⑧ ⊕ ⊕ ⊕ ⊕

OTHER BEVERAGES _____

SUPPLEMENTS/MEDICATIONS _____

DIGESTION/BOWEL MOVEMENTS _____

"WE NEVER KNOW HOW HIGH WE ARE
TILL WE ARE CALLED TO RISE; AND THEN,
IF WE ARE TRUE TO PLAN,
OUR STATURES TOUCH THE SKIES."
- EMILY DICKINSON

WHAT WOULD MAKE TODAY GREAT?

1. _____
2. _____
3. _____

MINDFULNESS

HOW DO I FEEL TODAY? _____
_____
_____
_____

MY MOOD IS...
- ☐ HAPPY
- ☐ FOCUSED
- ☐ ENERGETIC
- ☐ EXCITED
- ☐ SAD
- ☐ TIRED
- ☐ ANXIOUS
- ☐ ANGRY

FITNESS

EXERCISE _____
_____
_____
_____

I PRACTICED...
- ☐ MEDITATION
- ☐ LOVING SELF-TALK
- ☐ DEEP BREATHING

RATE MY...

- ENERGY LEVEL ☆☆☆
- SELF-CARE ☆☆☆
- HUNGER/CRAVINGS ☆☆☆
- RELATIONSHIP WITH FOOD & EXERCISE ☆☆☆

ONE THING I WOULD LIKE TO KEEP WORKING ON _____
_____
_____

3 THINGS I AM GRATEFUL FOR TODAY

1. _____
2. _____
3. _____

# OF STEPS	% BODY FAT	WEIGHT

Tuesday
WEEK 4

___/___/___

NUTRITION

	PROTEIN	STARCH	FRUIT	VEGETABLES	FATS
BREAKFAST 🕐					
MORNING SNACK 🕐					
LUNCH 🕐					
AFTERNOON SNACK 🕐					
DINNER 🕐					
EVENING SNACK 🕐					
TOTALS					

WATER 💧 ② ③ ④ ⑤ ⑥ ⑦ ⑧ ⊕ ⊕ ⊕ ⊕

OTHER BEVERAGES _____

SUPPLEMENTS/MEDICATIONS _____

DIGESTION/BOWEL MOVEMENTS _____

> "EARLY TO BED AND EARLY TO RISE MAKES A MAN HEALTHY, WEALTHY, AND WISE."
> - BENJAMIN FRANKLIN

WHAT WOULD MAKE TODAY GREAT?

1. _____
2. _____
3. _____

MINDFULNESS

HOW DO I FEEL TODAY? _____
_____
_____
_____

MY MOOD IS...

- ☐ HAPPY
- ☐ FOCUSED
- ☐ ENERGETIC
- ☐ EXCITED
- ☐ SAD
- ☐ TIRED
- ☐ ANXIOUS
- ☐ ANGRY

FITNESS

EXERCISE _____
_____
_____
_____

I PRACTICED...

- ☐ MEDITATION
- ☐ LOVING SELF-TALK
- ☐ DEEP BREATHING

RATE MY...

- ENERGY LEVEL ☆☆☆
- SELF-CARE ☆☆☆
- HUNGER/CRAVINGS ☆☆☆
- RELATIONSHIP WITH FOOD & EXERCISE ☆☆☆

ONE THING I WOULD LIKE TO KEEP WORKING ON _____
_____
_____

3 THINGS I AM GRATEFUL FOR TODAY

1. _____
2. _____
3. _____

# OF STEPS	% BODY FAT	WEIGHT

Wednesday ___/___/___
WEEK 4

NUTRITION

	PROTEIN	STARCH	FRUIT	VEGETABLES	FATS
BREAKFAST 🕐					
MORNING SNACK 🕐					
LUNCH 🕐					
AFTERNOON SNACK 🕐					
DINNER 🕐					
EVENING SNACK 🕐					
TOTALS					

WATER 💧 2 3 4 5 6 7 8 ⊕ ⊕ ⊕ ⊕

OTHER BEVERAGES _____

SUPPLEMENTS/MEDICATIONS _____

DIGESTION/BOWEL MOVEMENTS _____

"IF YOU WANT SOMETHING YOU'VE NEVER HAD, YOU MUST BE WILLING TO DO SOMETHING YOU'VE NEVER DONE."
- UNKNOWN

WHAT WOULD MAKE TODAY GREAT?

1. _____
2. _____
3. _____

MINDFULNESS

HOW DO I FEEL TODAY? _____
_____
_____
_____

MY MOOD IS...

- ☐ HAPPY
- ☐ SAD
- ☐ FOCUSED
- ☐ TIRED
- ☐ ENERGETIC
- ☐ ANXIOUS
- ☐ EXCITED
- ☐ ANGRY

I PRACTICED...

- ☐ MEDITATION
- ☐ LOVING SELF-TALK
- ☐ DEEP BREATHING

FITNESS

EXERCISE _____
_____
_____
_____

RATE MY...

- ENERGY LEVEL ☆☆☆
- SELF-CARE ☆☆☆
- HUNGER/CRAVINGS ☆☆☆
- RELATIONSHIP WITH FOOD & EXERCISE ☆☆☆

ONE THING I WOULD LIKE TO KEEP WORKING ON _____
_____
_____

3 THINGS I AM GRATEFUL FOR TODAY

1. _____
2. _____
3. _____

| # OF STEPS | | % BODY FAT | | WEIGHT | |

Thursday
WEEK 4

___/___/___

NUTRITION

	PROTEIN	STARCH	FRUIT	VEGETABLES	FATS
BREAKFAST 🕐					
MORNING SNACK 🕐					
LUNCH 🕐					
AFTERNOON SNACK 🕐					
DINNER 🕐					
EVENING SNACK 🕐					
TOTALS					

WATER 💧 ② ③ ④ ⑤ ⑥ ⑦ ⑧ ⊕ ⊕ ⊕ ⊕

OTHER BEVERAGES _____

SUPPLEMENTS/MEDICATIONS _____

DIGESTION/BOWEL MOVEMENTS _____

> "WHEN YOU ARISE IN THE MORNING, THINK OF WHAT A PRECIOUS PRIVILEGE IT IS TO BE ALIVE - TO BREATHE, TO THINK, TO ENJOY, TO LOVE."
> - MARCUS AURELIUS

WHAT WOULD MAKE TODAY GREAT?

1. _____
2. _____
3. _____

MINDFULNESS

HOW DO I FEEL TODAY? _____
_____
_____
_____

MY MOOD IS...

- ☐ HAPPY
- ☐ FOCUSED
- ☐ ENERGETIC
- ☐ EXCITED
- ☐ SAD
- ☐ TIRED
- ☐ ANXIOUS
- ☐ ANGRY

FITNESS

EXERCISE _____
_____
_____
_____

I PRACTICED...

- ☐ MEDITATION
- ☐ LOVING SELF-TALK
- ☐ DEEP BREATHING

RATE MY...

- ENERGY LEVEL ★ ★ ★
- SELF-CARE ★ ★ ★
- HUNGER/CRAVINGS ★ ★ ★
- RELATIONSHIP WITH FOOD & EXERCISE ★ ★ ★

ONE THING I WOULD LIKE TO KEEP WORKING ON _____
_____
_____

3 THINGS I AM GRATEFUL FOR TODAY

1. _____
2. _____
3. _____

# OF STEPS		% BODY FAT		WEIGHT	

Friday
WEEK 4

___/___/___

NUTRITION

		PROTEIN	STARCH	FRUIT	VEGETABLES	FATS
BREAKFAST 🕐						
MORNING SNACK 🕐						
LUNCH 🕐						
AFTERNOON SNACK 🕐						
DINNER 🕐						
EVENING SNACK 🕐						
TOTALS						

WATER 🍊 2 3 4 5 6 7 8 ⊕ ⊕ ⊕ ⊕

OTHER BEVERAGES _____

SUPPLEMENTS/MEDICATIONS _____

DIGESTION/BOWEL MOVEMENTS _____

"BELIEVE YOU CAN, AND YOU'RE HALFWAY THERE."
- THEODORE ROOSEVELT

WHAT WOULD MAKE TODAY GREAT?

1. _____
2. _____
3. _____

MINDFULNESS

HOW DO I FEEL TODAY? _____
_____
_____
_____

MY MOOD IS...

- ☐ HAPPY
- ☐ FOCUSED
- ☐ ENERGETIC
- ☐ EXCITED
- ☐ SAD
- ☐ TIRED
- ☐ ANXIOUS
- ☐ ANGRY

FITNESS

EXERCISE _____
_____
_____
_____

I PRACTICED...

- ☐ MEDITATION
- ☐ LOVING SELF-TALK
- ☐ DEEP BREATHING

RATE MY...

- ENERGY LEVEL ☆☆☆
- SELF-CARE ☆☆☆
- HUNGER/CRAVINGS ☆☆☆
- RELATIONSHIP WITH FOOD & EXERCISE ☆☆☆

ONE THING I WOULD LIKE TO KEEP WORKING ON _____
_____
_____

3 THINGS I AM GRATEFUL FOR TODAY

1. _____
2. _____
3. _____

☐ RECORD BODY MEASUREMENTS | # OF STEPS ____ | % BODY FAT ____ | WEIGHT ____

saturday
WEEK 4

___/___/___

NUTRITION

	PROTEIN	STARCH	FRUIT	VEGETABLES	FATS
BREAKFAST 🕐					
MORNING SNACK 🕐					
LUNCH 🕐					
AFTERNOON SNACK 🕐					
DINNER 🕐					
EVENING SNACK 🕐					
TOTALS					

WATER 💧 2 3 4 5 6 7 8 ➕ ➕ ➕ ➕

OTHER BEVERAGES _____

SUPPLEMENTS/MEDICATIONS _____

DIGESTION/BOWEL MOVEMENTS _____

> "KNOWING IS NOT ENOUGH; WE MUST APPLY.
> WILLING IS NOT ENOUGH; WE MUST DO."
> - JOHANN WOLFGANG VON GOETHE

WHAT WOULD MAKE TODAY GREAT?

1. _____
2. _____
3. _____

MINDFULNESS

HOW DO I FEEL TODAY? _____
_____
_____
_____

MY MOOD IS...

- ☐ HAPPY
- ☐ FOCUSED
- ☐ ENERGETIC
- ☐ EXCITED
- ☐ SAD
- ☐ TIRED
- ☐ ANXIOUS
- ☐ ANGRY

FITNESS

EXERCISE _____
_____
_____
_____

I PRACTICED...

- ☐ MEDITATION
- ☐ LOVING SELF-TALK
- ☐ DEEP BREATHING

RATE MY...

- ENERGY LEVEL ☆☆☆☆
- SELF-CARE ☆☆☆☆
- HUNGER/CRAVINGS ☆☆☆☆
- RELATIONSHIP WITH FOOD & EXERCISE ☆☆☆☆

ONE THING I WOULD LIKE TO KEEP WORKING ON _____
_____
_____

3 THINGS I AM GRATEFUL FOR TODAY

1. _____
2. _____
3. _____

# OF STEPS	% BODY FAT	WEIGHT

Sunday
WEEK 4

___/___/___

NUTRITION

	PROTEIN	STARCH	FRUIT	VEGETABLES	FATS
BREAKFAST 🕐					
MORNING SNACK 🕐					
LUNCH 🕐					
AFTERNOON SNACK 🕐					
DINNER 🕐					
EVENING SNACK 🕐					
TOTALS					

WATER 💧 ② ③ ④ ⑤ ⑥ ⑦ ⑧ ⊕ ⊕ ⊕

OTHER BEVERAGES _____

SUPPLEMENTS/MEDICATIONS _____

DIGESTION/BOWEL MOVEMENTS _____

**ASK YOURSELF TODAY:
HOW CAN I LEVEL-UP MY ROUTINE THIS WEEK?**

WHAT WOULD MAKE TODAY GREAT?

1. _____
2. _____
3. _____

MINDFULNESS

HOW DO I FEEL TODAY? _____
_____
_____
_____

MY MOOD IS...

- ☐ HAPPY
- ☐ FOCUSED
- ☐ ENERGETIC
- ☐ EXCITED
- ☐ SAD
- ☐ TIRED
- ☐ ANXIOUS
- ☐ ANGRY

FITNESS

EXERCISE _____
_____
_____

I PRACTICED...

- ☐ MEDITATION
- ☐ LOVING SELF-TALK
- ☐ DEEP BREATHING

RATE MY...

- ENERGY LEVEL ☆ ☆ ☆
- SELF-CARE ☆ ☆ ☆
- HUNGER/CRAVINGS ☆ ☆ ☆
- RELATIONSHIP WITH FOOD & EXERCISE ☆ ☆ ☆

3 THINGS I AM GRATEFUL FOR TODAY

1. _____
2. _____
3. _____

ONE THING I WOULD LIKE TO KEEP WORKING ON _____
_____
_____

# OF STEPS	% BODY FAT	WEIGHT

I AM...

STRONG

Week 5

Week 5 GOALS

GOALS FOR THIS WEEK

1. _____
   _____

2. _____
   _____

3. _____
   _____

EXERCISE PLAN

MONDAY _____
TUESDAY _____
WEDNESDAY _____
THURSDAY _____
FRIDAY _____
SATURDAY _____
SUNDAY _____

Week 5
MEAL PLAN & GROCERY LIST

MONDAY
- B
- L
- D
- SNACKS

TUESDAY
- B
- L
- D
- SNACKS

WEDNESDAY
- B
- L
- D
- SNACKS

THURSDAY
- B
- L
- D
- SNACKS

FRIDAY
- B
- L
- D
- SNACKS

SATURDAY
- B
- L
- D
- SNACKS

SUNDAY
- B
- L
- D
- SNACKS

GROCERY LIST

Monday
WEEK 5

___/___/___

NUTRITION

	PROTEIN	STARCH	FRUIT	VEGETABLES	FATS
BREAKFAST					
MORNING SNACK					
LUNCH					
AFTERNOON SNACK					
DINNER					
EVENING SNACK					
TOTALS					

WATER ① ② ③ ④ ⑤ ⑥ ⑦ ⑧ ⊕ ⊕ ⊕ ⊕

OTHER BEVERAGES _____

SUPPLEMENTS/MEDICATIONS _____

DIGESTION/BOWEL MOVEMENTS _____

> "THERE ARE SEVEN DAYS IN THE WEEK AND SOMEDAY ISN'T ONE OF THEM."
> - UNKNOWN

WHAT WOULD MAKE TODAY GREAT?

1. _____
2. _____
3. _____

MINDFULNESS

HOW DO I FEEL TODAY? _____

_____
_____
_____

MY MOOD IS...

- ☐ HAPPY
- ☐ FOCUSED
- ☐ ENERGETIC
- ☐ EXCITED
- ☐ SAD
- ☐ TIRED
- ☐ ANXIOUS
- ☐ ANGRY

I PRACTICED...

- ☐ MEDITATION
- ☐ LOVING SELF-TALK
- ☐ DEEP BREATHING

FITNESS

EXERCISE _____
_____
_____
_____

RATE MY...

- ENERGY LEVEL ☆☆☆
- SELF-CARE ☆☆☆
- HUNGER/CRAVINGS ☆☆☆
- RELATIONSHIP WITH FOOD & EXERCISE ☆☆☆

ONE THING I WOULD LIKE TO KEEP WORKING ON _____
_____
_____

3 THINGS I AM GRATEFUL FOR TODAY

1. _____
2. _____
3. _____

# OF STEPS	% BODY FAT	WEIGHT

Tuesday
WEEK 5

___/___/___

NUTRITION

	PROTEIN	STARCH	FRUIT	VEGETABLES	FATS
BREAKFAST 🕐					
MORNING SNACK 🕐					
LUNCH 🕐					
AFTERNOON SNACK 🕐					
DINNER 🕐					
EVENING SNACK 🕐					
TOTALS					

WATER 💧 ② ③ ④ ⑤ ⑥ ⑦ ⑧ ⊕ ⊕ ⊕ ⊕

OTHER BEVERAGES _____

SUPPLEMENTS/MEDICATIONS _____

DIGESTION/BOWEL MOVEMENTS _____

YOU ARE CAPABLE OF FAR MORE
THAN YOU KNOW.

WHAT WOULD MAKE TODAY GREAT?

1. _____
2. _____
3. _____

MINDFULNESS

HOW DO I FEEL TODAY? _____
_____
_____
_____

MY MOOD IS...

☐ HAPPY ☐ SAD
☐ FOCUSED ☐ TIRED
☐ ENERGETIC ☐ ANXIOUS
☐ EXCITED ☐ ANGRY

FITNESS

EXERCISE _____
_____
_____
_____

I PRACTICED...

☐ MEDITATION
☐ LOVING SELF-TALK
☐ DEEP BREATHING

RATE MY...

ENERGY LEVEL ★ ★ ★
SELF-CARE ★ ★ ★
HUNGER/CRAVINGS ★ ★ ★
RELATIONSHIP WITH FOOD & EXERCISE ★ ★ ★

ONE THING I WOULD LIKE TO KEEP WORKING ON _____
_____
_____

3 THINGS I AM GRATEFUL FOR TODAY

1. _____
2. _____
3. _____

| # OF STEPS | | % BODY FAT | | WEIGHT | |

Wednesday ___/___/___
WEEK 5

NUTRITION

	PROTEIN	STARCH	FRUIT	VEGETABLES	FATS
BREAKFAST 🕐					
MORNING SNACK 🕐					
LUNCH 🕐					
AFTERNOON SNACK 🕐					
DINNER 🕐					
EVENING SNACK 🕐					
TOTALS					

WATER 🍊 ② ③ ④ ⑤ ⑥ ⑦ ⑧ ⊕ ⊕ ⊕

OTHER BEVERAGES _____

SUPPLEMENTS/MEDICATIONS _____

DIGESTION/BOWEL MOVEMENTS _____

*"IF YOU CANNOT DO GREAT THINGS,
DO SMALL THINGS IN A GREAT WAY."
- NAPOLEON HILL*

WHAT WOULD MAKE TODAY GREAT?

1. _____
2. _____
3. _____

MINDFULNESS

HOW DO I FEEL TODAY? _____

_____

_____

MY MOOD IS...

- ☐ HAPPY
- ☐ FOCUSED
- ☐ ENERGETIC
- ☐ EXCITED
- ☐ SAD
- ☐ TIRED
- ☐ ANXIOUS
- ☐ ANGRY

I PRACTICED...

- ☐ MEDITATION
- ☐ LOVING SELF-TALK
- ☐ DEEP BREATHING

FITNESS

EXERCISE _____

_____

_____

_____

RATE MY...

- ENERGY LEVEL ☆☆☆
- SELF-CARE ☆☆☆
- HUNGER/CRAVINGS ☆☆☆
- RELATIONSHIP WITH FOOD & EXERCISE ☆☆☆

ONE THING I WOULD LIKE TO KEEP WORKING ON _____

_____

_____

3 THINGS I AM GRATEFUL FOR TODAY

1. _____
2. _____
3. _____

# OF STEPS	% BODY FAT	WEIGHT

Thursday

WEEK 5

___/___/___

NUTRITION

		PROTEIN	STARCH	FRUIT	VEGETABLES	FATS
BREAKFAST 🕐						
MORNING SNACK 🕐						
LUNCH 🕐						
AFTERNOON SNACK 🕐						
DINNER 🕐						
EVENING SNACK 🕐						
TOTALS						

WATER 💧 ② ③ ④ ⑤ ⑥ ⑦ ⑧ ⊕ ⊕ ⊕ ⊕

OTHER BEVERAGES _____

SUPPLEMENTS/MEDICATIONS _____

DIGESTION/BOWEL MOVEMENTS _____

> "I SHALL NOT WASTE MY DAYS IN TRYING TO PROLONG THEM.
> I SHALL USE MY TIME."
> - JACK LONDON

WHAT WOULD MAKE TODAY GREAT?

1. _____
2. _____
3. _____

MINDFULNESS

HOW DO I FEEL TODAY? _____
_____
_____
_____

MY MOOD IS...

- ☐ HAPPY
- ☐ FOCUSED
- ☐ ENERGETIC
- ☐ EXCITED
- ☐ SAD
- ☐ TIRED
- ☐ ANXIOUS
- ☐ ANGRY

FITNESS

EXERCISE _____
_____
_____
_____

I PRACTICED...

- ☐ MEDITATION
- ☐ LOVING SELF-TALK
- ☐ DEEP BREATHING

RATE MY...

- ENERGY LEVEL ☆☆☆
- SELF-CARE ☆☆☆
- HUNGER/CRAVINGS ☆☆☆
- RELATIONSHIP WITH FOOD & EXERCISE ☆☆☆

ONE THING I WOULD LIKE TO KEEP WORKING ON _____
_____
_____

3 THINGS I AM GRATEFUL FOR TODAY

1. _____
2. _____
3. _____

| # OF STEPS | | % BODY FAT | | WEIGHT | |

Friday
WEEK 5

___/___/___

NUTRITION

		PROTEIN	STARCH	FRUIT	VEGETABLES	FATS
BREAKFAST 🕐						
MORNING SNACK 🕐						
LUNCH 🕐						
AFTERNOON SNACK 🕐						
DINNER 🕐						
EVENING SNACK 🕐						
TOTALS						

WATER 🍊 ② ③ ④ ⑤ ⑥ ⑦ ⑧ ⊕ ⊕ ⊕ ⊕

OTHER BEVERAGES _____

SUPPLEMENTS/MEDICATIONS _____

DIGESTION/BOWEL MOVEMENTS _____

> "IF WE ARE WALKING IN THE RIGHT DIRECTION,
> ALL WE HAVE TO DO IS KEEP WALKING."
> - UNKNOWN

WHAT WOULD MAKE TODAY GREAT?

1. _____
2. _____
3. _____

MINDFULNESS

HOW DO I FEEL TODAY? _____

_____

_____

_____

MY MOOD IS...

- ☐ HAPPY
- ☐ FOCUSED
- ☐ ENERGETIC
- ☐ EXCITED
- ☐ SAD
- ☐ TIRED
- ☐ ANXIOUS
- ☐ ANGRY

FITNESS

EXERCISE _____

_____

_____

_____

I PRACTICED...

- ☐ MEDITATION
- ☐ LOVING SELF-TALK
- ☐ DEEP BREATHING

RATE MY...

- ENERGY LEVEL ☆ ☆ ☆
- SELF-CARE ☆ ☆ ☆
- HUNGER/CRAVINGS ☆ ☆ ☆
- RELATIONSHIP WITH FOOD & EXERCISE ☆ ☆ ☆

ONE THING I WOULD LIKE TO KEEP WORKING ON _____

_____

_____

3 THINGS I AM GRATEFUL FOR TODAY

1. _____
2. _____
3. _____

# OF STEPS		% BODY FAT		WEIGHT	

saturday

WEEK 5   __/__/__

NUTRITION

		PROTEIN	STARCH	FRUIT	VEGETABLES	FATS
BREAKFAST 🕐						
MORNING SNACK 🕐						
LUNCH 🕐						
AFTERNOON SNACK 🕐						
DINNER 🕐						
EVENING SNACK 🕐						
TOTALS						

WATER 💧 ② ③ ④ ⑤ ⑥ ⑦ ⑧ ⊕ ⊕ ⊕ ⊕

OTHER BEVERAGES _____

SUPPLEMENTS/MEDICATIONS _____

DIGESTION/BOWEL MOVEMENTS _____

> "ONCE YOU MAKE A DECISION, THE UNIVERSE CONSPIRES TO MAKE IT HAPPEN."
> - RALPH WALDO EMERSON

WHAT WOULD MAKE TODAY GREAT?

1. _____
2. _____
3. _____

MINDFULNESS

HOW DO I FEEL TODAY? _____
_____
_____
_____

MY MOOD IS...
- ☐ HAPPY
- ☐ FOCUSED
- ☐ ENERGETIC
- ☐ EXCITED
- ☐ SAD
- ☐ TIRED
- ☐ ANXIOUS
- ☐ ANGRY

I PRACTICED...
- ☐ MEDITATION
- ☐ LOVING SELF-TALK
- ☐ DEEP BREATHING

FITNESS

EXERCISE _____
_____
_____
_____

RATE MY...
- ENERGY LEVEL ☆ ☆ ☆
- SELF-CARE ☆ ☆ ☆
- HUNGER/CRAVINGS ☆ ☆ ☆
- RELATIONSHIP WITH FOOD & EXERCISE ☆ ☆ ☆

ONE THING I WOULD LIKE TO KEEP WORKING ON _____
_____
_____

3 THINGS I AM GRATEFUL FOR TODAY

1. _____
2. _____
3. _____

| # OF STEPS | | % BODY FAT | | WEIGHT | |

Sunday
WEEK 5

___/___/___

NUTRITION

		PROTEIN	STARCH	FRUIT	VEGETABLES	FATS
BREAKFAST 🕐						
MORNING SNACK 🕐						
LUNCH 🕐						
AFTERNOON SNACK 🕐						
DINNER 🕐						
EVENING SNACK 🕐						
TOTALS						

WATER 🍊 ② ③ ④ ⑤ ⑥ ⑦ ⑧ ⊕ ⊕ ⊕ ⊕

OTHER BEVERAGES _____

SUPPLEMENTS/MEDICATIONS _____

DIGESTION/BOWEL MOVEMENTS _____

ASK YOURSELF TODAY:
WHAT TYPE OF MOVEMENT MAKES MY
BODY FEEL BEST?

WHAT WOULD MAKE TODAY GREAT?

1. _____
2. _____
3. _____

MINDFULNESS

HOW DO I FEEL TODAY? _____
_____
_____
_____

MY MOOD IS...

- ☐ HAPPY
- ☐ FOCUSED
- ☐ ENERGETIC
- ☐ EXCITED
- ☐ SAD
- ☐ TIRED
- ☐ ANXIOUS
- ☐ ANGRY

FITNESS

EXERCISE _____
_____
_____
_____

I PRACTICED...

- ☐ MEDITATION
- ☐ LOVING SELF-TALK
- ☐ DEEP BREATHING

RATE MY...

- ENERGY LEVEL ☆☆☆
- SELF-CARE ☆☆☆
- HUNGER/CRAVINGS ☆☆☆
- RELATIONSHIP WITH FOOD & EXERCISE ☆☆☆

ONE THING I WOULD LIKE TO KEEP WORKING ON _____
_____
_____

3 THINGS I AM GRATEFUL FOR TODAY

1. _____
2. _____
3. _____

| # OF STEPS | | % BODY FAT | | WEIGHT | |

I AM...

POWERFUL

Week 6

Week 6 GOALS

GOALS FOR THIS WEEK

① _____
_____
_____

② _____
_____
_____

③ _____
_____
_____

EXERCISE PLAN

MONDAY _____
TUESDAY _____
WEDNESDAY _____
THURSDAY _____
FRIDAY _____
SATURDAY _____
SUNDAY _____

Week 6
MEAL PLAN & GROCERY LIST

MONDAY
- (B)
- (L)
- (D)

SNACKS

TUESDAY
- (B)
- (L)
- (D)

SNACKS

WEDNESDAY
- (B)
- (L)
- (D)

SNACKS

THURSDAY
- (B)
- (L)
- (D)

SNACKS

FRIDAY
- (B)
- (L)
- (D)

SNACKS

SATURDAY
- (B)
- (L)
- (D)

SNACKS

SUNDAY
- (B)
- (L)
- (D)

SNACKS

GROCERY LIST

Monday
WEEK 6

___/___/___

NUTRITION

	PROTEIN	STARCH	FRUIT	VEGETABLES	FATS
BREAKFAST 🕐					
MORNING SNACK 🕐					
LUNCH 🕐					
AFTERNOON SNACK 🕐					
DINNER 🕐					
EVENING SNACK 🕐					
TOTALS					

WATER 💧 2 3 4 5 6 7 8 ⊕ ⊕ ⊕ ⊕

OTHER BEVERAGES _____

SUPPLEMENTS/MEDICATIONS _____

DIGESTION/BOWEL MOVEMENTS _____

> "IF YOU TAKE CARE OF THE MINUTES
> THE YEARS WILL TAKE CARE OF THEMSELVES."
> - ANCIENT TIBETAN PROVERB

WHAT WOULD MAKE TODAY GREAT?

1. _____
2. _____
3. _____

MINDFULNESS

HOW DO I FEEL TODAY? _____

_____
_____
_____

MY MOOD IS...

- ☐ HAPPY
- ☐ FOCUSED
- ☐ ENERGETIC
- ☐ EXCITED
- ☐ SAD
- ☐ TIRED
- ☐ ANXIOUS
- ☐ ANGRY

I PRACTICED...

- ☐ MEDITATION
- ☐ LOVING SELF-TALK
- ☐ DEEP BREATHING

FITNESS

EXERCISE _____
_____
_____
_____

RATE MY...

- ENERGY LEVEL ☆ ☆ ☆
- SELF-CARE ☆ ☆ ☆
- HUNGER/CRAVINGS ☆ ☆ ☆
- RELATIONSHIP WITH FOOD & EXERCISE ☆ ☆ ☆

ONE THING I WOULD LIKE TO KEEP WORKING ON _____
_____
_____

3 THINGS I AM GRATEFUL FOR TODAY

1. _____
2. _____
3. _____

| # OF STEPS | | % BODY FAT | | WEIGHT | |

Tuesday
WEEK 6

___/___/___

NUTRITION

	PROTEIN	STARCH	FRUIT	VEGETABLES	FATS
BREAKFAST 🕐					
MORNING SNACK 🕐					
LUNCH 🕐					
AFTERNOON SNACK 🕐					
DINNER 🕐					
EVENING SNACK 🕐					
TOTALS					

WATER 💧 ② ③ ④ ⑤ ⑥ ⑦ ⑧ ➕ ➕ ➕

OTHER BEVERAGES _____

SUPPLEMENTS/MEDICATIONS _____

DIGESTION/BOWEL MOVEMENTS _____

"WE AIM ABOVE THE MARK TO HIT THE MARK."
- RALPH WALDO EMERSON

WHAT WOULD MAKE TODAY GREAT?

1. _____
2. _____
3. _____

MINDFULNESS

HOW DO I FEEL TODAY? _____
_____
_____
_____

MY MOOD IS...

- ☐ HAPPY
- ☐ FOCUSED
- ☐ ENERGETIC
- ☐ EXCITED
- ☐ SAD
- ☐ TIRED
- ☐ ANXIOUS
- ☐ ANGRY

I PRACTICED...

- ☐ MEDITATION
- ☐ LOVING SELF-TALK
- ☐ DEEP BREATHING

FITNESS

EXERCISE _____
_____
_____
_____

RATE MY...

- ENERGY LEVEL ☆ ☆ ☆
- SELF-CARE ☆ ☆ ☆
- HUNGER/CRAVINGS ☆ ☆ ☆
- RELATIONSHIP WITH FOOD & EXERCISE ☆ ☆ ☆

ONE THING I WOULD LIKE TO KEEP WORKING ON _____
_____
_____

3 THINGS I AM GRATEFUL FOR TODAY

1. _____
2. _____
3. _____

# OF STEPS		% BODY FAT		WEIGHT	

Wednesday ___/___/___
WEEK 6

NUTRITION

		PROTEIN	STARCH	FRUIT	VEGETABLES	FATS
BREAKFAST 🕐						
MORNING SNACK 🕐						
LUNCH 🕐						
AFTERNOON SNACK 🕐						
DINNER 🕐						
EVENING SNACK 🕐						
TOTALS						

WATER 🍋 ② ③ ④ ⑤ ⑥ ⑦ ⑧ ⊕ ⊕ ⊕ ⊕

OTHER BEVERAGES _____

SUPPLEMENTS/MEDICATIONS _____

DIGESTION/BOWEL MOVEMENTS _____

"A SMOOTH SEA NEVER MADE A SKILLFUL SAILOR."
- PROVERB

WHAT WOULD MAKE TODAY GREAT?

① _____
② _____
③ _____

MINDFULNESS

HOW DO I FEEL TODAY? _____
_____
_____
_____

MY MOOD IS...

- ☐ HAPPY
- ☐ FOCUSED
- ☐ ENERGETIC
- ☐ EXCITED
- ☐ SAD
- ☐ TIRED
- ☐ ANXIOUS
- ☐ ANGRY

I PRACTICED...

- ☐ MEDITATION
- ☐ LOVING SELF-TALK
- ☐ DEEP BREATHING

FITNESS

EXERCISE _____
_____
_____
_____

RATE MY...

- ENERGY LEVEL ☆☆☆
- SELF-CARE ☆☆☆
- HUNGER/CRAVINGS ☆☆☆
- RELATIONSHIP WITH FOOD & EXERCISE ☆☆☆

ONE THING I WOULD LIKE TO KEEP WORKING ON _____
_____
_____

3 THINGS I AM GRATEFUL FOR TODAY

① _____
② _____
③ _____

| # OF STEPS | | % BODY FAT | | WEIGHT | |

Thursday
WEEK 6

___/___/___

NUTRITION

	PROTEIN	STARCH	FRUIT	VEGETABLES	FATS
BREAKFAST 🕐					
MORNING SNACK 🕐					
LUNCH 🕐					
AFTERNOON SNACK 🕐					
DINNER 🕐					
EVENING SNACK 🕐					
TOTALS					

WATER 💧 ② ③ ④ ⑤ ⑥ ⑦ ⑧ ⊕ ⊕ ⊕ ⊕

OTHER BEVERAGES _____

SUPPLEMENTS/MEDICATIONS _____

DIGESTION/BOWEL MOVEMENTS _____

> "ONE MUST DARE TO BE HAPPY."
> - GERTRUDE STEIN

WHAT WOULD MAKE TODAY GREAT?

1. _____
2. _____
3. _____

MINDFULNESS

HOW DO I FEEL TODAY? _____
_____
_____
_____

MY MOOD IS...
- ☐ HAPPY
- ☐ FOCUSED
- ☐ ENERGETIC
- ☐ EXCITED
- ☐ SAD
- ☐ TIRED
- ☐ ANXIOUS
- ☐ ANGRY

I PRACTICED...
- ☐ MEDITATION
- ☐ LOVING SELF-TALK
- ☐ DEEP BREATHING

FITNESS

EXERCISE _____
_____
_____
_____

RATE MY...
- ENERGY LEVEL ☆ ☆ ☆
- SELF-CARE ☆ ☆ ☆
- HUNGER/CRAVINGS ☆ ☆ ☆
- RELATIONSHIP WITH FOOD & EXERCISE ☆ ☆ ☆

ONE THING I WOULD LIKE TO KEEP WORKING ON _____
_____
_____

3 THINGS I AM GRATEFUL FOR TODAY

1. _____
2. _____
3. _____

| # OF STEPS | | % BODY FAT | | WEIGHT | |

Friday
WEEK 6

___/___/___

NUTRITION

	PROTEIN	STARCH	FRUIT	VEGETABLES	FATS
BREAKFAST 🕐					
MORNING SNACK 🕐					
LUNCH 🕐					
AFTERNOON SNACK 🕐					
DINNER 🕐					
EVENING SNACK 🕐					
TOTALS					

WATER 🍋 ② ③ ④ ⑤ ⑥ ⑦ ⑧ ⊕ ⊕ ⊕ ⊕

OTHER BEVERAGES _____

SUPPLEMENTS/MEDICATIONS _____

DIGESTION/BOWEL MOVEMENTS _____

"IF YOU HAVE MORE THAN THREE PRIORITIES, THEN YOU DON'T HAVE ANY."
- JIM COLLINS

WHAT WOULD MAKE TODAY GREAT?

1. _____
2. _____
3. _____

MINDFULNESS

HOW DO I FEEL TODAY? _____
_____
_____
_____

MY MOOD IS...

- ☐ HAPPY
- ☐ FOCUSED
- ☐ ENERGETIC
- ☐ EXCITED
- ☐ SAD
- ☐ TIRED
- ☐ ANXIOUS
- ☐ ANGRY

I PRACTICED...

- ☐ MEDITATION
- ☐ LOVING SELF-TALK
- ☐ DEEP BREATHING

FITNESS

EXERCISE _____
_____
_____
_____

RATE MY...

- ENERGY LEVEL ☆☆☆
- SELF-CARE ☆☆☆
- HUNGER/CRAVINGS ☆☆☆
- RELATIONSHIP WITH FOOD & EXERCISE ☆☆☆

ONE THING I WOULD LIKE TO KEEP WORKING ON _____
_____
_____

3 THINGS I AM GRATEFUL FOR TODAY

1. _____
2. _____
3. _____

☐ RECORD BODY MEASUREMENTS | # OF STEPS ___ | % BODY FAT ___ | WEIGHT ___

saturday
WEEK 6

___/___/___

NUTRITION

	PROTEIN	STARCH	FRUIT	VEGETABLES	FATS
BREAKFAST 🕐					
MORNING SNACK 🕐					
LUNCH 🕐					
AFTERNOON SNACK 🕐					
DINNER 🕐					
EVENING SNACK 🕐					
TOTALS					

WATER 💧 ② ③ ④ ⑤ ⑥ ⑦ ⑧ ⊕ ⊕ ⊕ ⊕

OTHER BEVERAGES _____

SUPPLEMENTS/MEDICATIONS _____

DIGESTION/BOWEL MOVEMENTS _____

> "YOU CAN'T HELP SOMEONE UPHILL WITHOUT GETTING CLOSER TO THE TOP YOURSELF."
> - PROVERB

WHAT WOULD MAKE TODAY GREAT?

1. _____
2. _____
3. _____

MINDFULNESS

HOW DO I FEEL TODAY? _____
_____
_____
_____

MY MOOD IS...

- ☐ HAPPY
- ☐ FOCUSED
- ☐ ENERGETIC
- ☐ EXCITED
- ☐ SAD
- ☐ TIRED
- ☐ ANXIOUS
- ☐ ANGRY

FITNESS

EXERCISE _____
_____
_____
_____

I PRACTICED...

- ☐ MEDITATION
- ☐ LOVING SELF-TALK
- ☐ DEEP BREATHING

RATE MY...

- ENERGY LEVEL ☆☆☆☆☆
- SELF-CARE ☆☆☆☆☆
- HUNGER/CRAVINGS ☆☆☆☆☆
- RELATIONSHIP WITH FOOD & EXERCISE ☆☆☆☆☆

ONE THING I WOULD LIKE TO KEEP WORKING ON _____
_____
_____

3 THINGS I AM GRATEFUL FOR TODAY

1. _____
2. _____
3. _____

| # OF STEPS | | % BODY FAT | | WEIGHT | |

Sunday
WEEK 6

___/___/___

NUTRITION

	PROTEIN	STARCH	FRUIT	VEGETABLES	FATS
BREAKFAST 🕐					
MORNING SNACK 🕐					
LUNCH 🕐					
AFTERNOON SNACK 🕐					
DINNER 🕐					
EVENING SNACK 🕐					
TOTALS					

WATER 🍋 ② ③ ④ ⑤ ⑥ ⑦ ⑧ ⊕ ⊕ ⊕ ⊕

OTHER BEVERAGES _____

SUPPLEMENTS/MEDICATIONS _____

DIGESTION/BOWEL MOVEMENTS _____

**ASK YOURSELF TODAY:
WHAT DOES IT FEEL LIKE TO FEEL STRONG
IN MY BODY?**

WHAT WOULD MAKE TODAY GREAT?

1. _____
2. _____
3. _____

MINDFULNESS

HOW DO I FEEL TODAY? _____
_____
_____
_____

MY MOOD IS...

- ☐ HAPPY
- ☐ FOCUSED
- ☐ ENERGETIC
- ☐ EXCITED
- ☐ SAD
- ☐ TIRED
- ☐ ANXIOUS
- ☐ ANGRY

FITNESS

EXERCISE _____
_____
_____
_____

I PRACTICED...

- ☐ MEDITATION
- ☐ LOVING SELF-TALK
- ☐ DEEP BREATHING

RATE MY...

- ENERGY LEVEL ☆ ☆ ☆
- SELF-CARE ☆ ☆ ☆
- HUNGER/CRAVINGS ☆ ☆ ☆
- RELATIONSHIP WITH FOOD & EXERCISE ☆ ☆ ☆

ONE THING I WOULD LIKE TO KEEP WORKING ON _____
_____
_____

3 THINGS I AM GRATEFUL FOR TODAY

1. _____
2. _____
3. _____

# OF STEPS	% BODY FAT	WEIGHT

I AM...

VIBRANT

Week 7

Week 7 GOALS

GOALS FOR THIS WEEK

1. _____

2. _____

3. _____

EXERCISE PLAN

MONDAY _____
TUESDAY _____
WEDNESDAY _____
THURSDAY _____
FRIDAY _____
SATURDAY _____
SUNDAY _____

Week 7
MEAL PLAN & GROCERY LIST

MONDAY
- B
- L
- D

SNACKS

TUESDAY
- B
- L
- D

SNACKS

WEDNESDAY
- B
- L
- D

SNACKS

THURSDAY
- B
- L
- D

SNACKS

FRIDAY
- B
- L
- D

SNACKS

SATURDAY
- B
- L
- D

SNACKS

SUNDAY
- B
- L
- D

SNACKS

GROCERY LIST

Monday
WEEK 7

___/___/___

NUTRITION

		PROTEIN	STARCH	FRUIT	VEGETABLES	FATS
BREAKFAST 🕐						
MORNING SNACK 🕐						
LUNCH 🕐						
AFTERNOON SNACK 🕐						
DINNER 🕐						
EVENING SNACK 🕐						
TOTALS						

WATER 🍊 2 3 4 5 6 7 8 ➕ ➕ ➕

OTHER BEVERAGES _____

SUPPLEMENTS/MEDICATIONS _____

DIGESTION/BOWEL MOVEMENTS _____

"REPLACE FEAR OF THE UNKNOWN WITH CURIOUSITY."
- UNKNOWN

WHAT WOULD MAKE TODAY GREAT?

1. _____
   _____
2. _____
   _____
3. _____
   _____

MINDFULNESS

HOW DO I FEEL TODAY? _____
_____
_____
_____

MY MOOD IS...

- ☐ HAPPY
- ☐ FOCUSED
- ☐ ENERGETIC
- ☐ EXCITED
- ☐ SAD
- ☐ TIRED
- ☐ ANXIOUS
- ☐ ANGRY

I PRACTICED...

- ☐ MEDITATION
- ☐ LOVING SELF-TALK
- ☐ DEEP BREATHING

FITNESS

EXERCISE _____
_____
_____
_____

RATE MY...

ENERGY LEVEL	★ ★ ★
SELF-CARE	★ ★ ★
HUNGER/CRAVINGS	★ ★ ★
RELATIONSHIP WITH FOOD & EXERCISE	★ ★ ★

ONE THING I WOULD LIKE TO KEEP WORKING ON _____
_____
_____

3 THINGS I AM GRATEFUL FOR TODAY

1. _____
   _____
2. _____
   _____
3. _____
   _____

# OF STEPS		% BODY FAT		WEIGHT	

Tuesday
WEEK 7

___/___/___

NUTRITION

	PROTEIN	STARCH	FRUIT	VEGETABLES	FATS
BREAKFAST 🕐					
MORNING SNACK 🕐					
LUNCH 🕐					
AFTERNOON SNACK 🕐					
DINNER 🕐					
EVENING SNACK 🕐					
TOTALS					

WATER 💧 2 3 4 5 6 7 8 ⊕ ⊕ ⊕ ⊕

OTHER BEVERAGES _____

SUPPLEMENTS/MEDICATIONS _____

DIGESTION/BOWEL MOVEMENTS _____

> "OUR GREATEST GLORY IS, NOT IN NEVER FALLING,
> BUT IN RISING EVERY TIME WE FALL."
> - OLIVER GOLDSMITH

WHAT WOULD MAKE TODAY GREAT?

1. _____
2. _____
3. _____

MINDFULNESS

HOW DO I FEEL TODAY? _____
_____
_____

MY MOOD IS...

- ☐ HAPPY
- ☐ FOCUSED
- ☐ ENERGETIC
- ☐ EXCITED
- ☐ SAD
- ☐ TIRED
- ☐ ANXIOUS
- ☐ ANGRY

FITNESS

EXERCISE _____
_____
_____
_____

I PRACTICED...

- ☐ MEDITATION
- ☐ LOVING SELF-TALK
- ☐ DEEP BREATHING

RATE MY...

- ENERGY LEVEL ☆ ☆ ☆
- SELF-CARE ☆ ☆ ☆
- HUNGER/CRAVINGS ☆ ☆ ☆
- RELATIONSHIP WITH FOOD & EXERCISE ☆ ☆ ☆

ONE THING I WOULD LIKE TO KEEP WORKING ON _____
_____
_____

3 THINGS I AM GRATEFUL FOR TODAY

1. _____
2. _____
3. _____

| # OF STEPS | | % BODY FAT | | WEIGHT | |

Wednesday ___/___/___
WEEK 7

NUTRITION

		PROTEIN	STARCH	FRUIT	VEGETABLES	FATS
BREAKFAST 🕐						
MORNING SNACK 🕐						
LUNCH 🕐						
AFTERNOON SNACK 🕐						
DINNER 🕐						
EVENING SNACK 🕐						
TOTALS						

WATER 🍊 ② ③ ④ ⑤ ⑥ ⑦ ⑧ ⊕ ⊕ ⊕ ⊕

OTHER BEVERAGES _____

SUPPLEMENTS/MEDICATIONS _____

DIGESTION/BOWEL MOVEMENTS _____

> "BE CAREFUL WHAT BOXES YOU PUT YOURSELF INTO.
> YOU MAY BELONG IN A DIFFERENT BOX!"
> - JENNIFER ANTHONY

WHAT WOULD MAKE TODAY GREAT?

1. _____
2. _____
3. _____

MINDFULNESS

HOW DO I FEEL TODAY? _____
_____
_____
_____

MY MOOD IS...

- ☐ HAPPY
- ☐ FOCUSED
- ☐ ENERGETIC
- ☐ EXCITED
- ☐ SAD
- ☐ TIRED
- ☐ ANXIOUS
- ☐ ANGRY

FITNESS

EXERCISE _____
_____
_____
_____

I PRACTICED...

- ☐ MEDITATION
- ☐ LOVING SELF-TALK
- ☐ DEEP BREATHING

RATE MY...

- ENERGY LEVEL ☆ ☆ ☆
- SELF-CARE ☆ ☆ ☆
- HUNGER/CRAVINGS ☆ ☆ ☆
- RELATIONSHIP WITH FOOD & EXERCISE ☆ ☆ ☆

ONE THING I WOULD LIKE TO KEEP WORKING ON _____
_____
_____

3 THINGS I AM GRATEFUL FOR TODAY

1. _____
2. _____
3. _____

# OF STEPS		% BODY FAT		WEIGHT	

Thursday

WEEK 7

___/___/___

NUTRITION

	PROTEIN	STARCH	FRUIT	VEGETABLES	FATS
BREAKFAST 🕐					
MORNING SNACK 🕐					
LUNCH 🕐					
AFTERNOON SNACK 🕐					
DINNER 🕐					
EVENING SNACK 🕐					
TOTALS					

WATER 💧 2 3 4 5 6 7 8 ➕ ➕ ➕

OTHER BEVERAGES _____

SUPPLEMENTS/MEDICATIONS _____

DIGESTION/BOWEL MOVEMENTS _____

"I DWELL IN POSSIBILITY."
- EMILY DICKINSON

WHAT WOULD MAKE TODAY GREAT?

1. _____
2. _____
3. _____

MINDFULNESS

HOW DO I FEEL TODAY? _____

_____
_____
_____

MY MOOD IS...

- ☐ HAPPY
- ☐ FOCUSED
- ☐ ENERGETIC
- ☐ EXCITED
- ☐ SAD
- ☐ TIRED
- ☐ ANXIOUS
- ☐ ANGRY

FITNESS

EXERCISE _____

_____
_____
_____

I PRACTICED...

- ☐ MEDITATION
- ☐ LOVING SELF-TALK
- ☐ DEEP BREATHING

RATE MY...

- ENERGY LEVEL ☆☆☆
- SELF-CARE ☆☆☆
- HUNGER/CRAVINGS ☆☆☆
- RELATIONSHIP WITH FOOD & EXERCISE ☆☆☆

ONE THING I WOULD LIKE TO KEEP WORKING ON _____

_____

3 THINGS I AM GRATEFUL FOR TODAY

1. _____
2. _____
3. _____

# OF STEPS	% BODY FAT	WEIGHT

Friday
WEEK 7

___/___/___

NUTRITION

	PROTEIN	STARCH	FRUIT	VEGETABLES	FATS
BREAKFAST					
MORNING SNACK					
LUNCH					
AFTERNOON SNACK					
DINNER					
EVENING SNACK					
TOTALS					

WATER ◯ 2 3 4 5 6 7 8 ⊕ ⊕ ⊕ ⊕

OTHER BEVERAGES _____

SUPPLEMENTS/MEDICATIONS _____

DIGESTION/BOWEL MOVEMENTS _____

> "WE HAVE TO CONTINUALLY BE JUMPING OFF CLIFFS AND
> DEVELOPING OUR WINGS ON THE WAY DOWN."
> - KURT VONNEGUT

WHAT WOULD MAKE TODAY GREAT?

1. _____
2. _____
3. _____

MINDFULNESS

HOW DO I FEEL TODAY? _____

_____
_____
_____

MY MOOD IS...

- ☐ HAPPY
- ☐ FOCUSED
- ☐ ENERGETIC
- ☐ EXCITED
- ☐ SAD
- ☐ TIRED
- ☐ ANXIOUS
- ☐ ANGRY

FITNESS

EXERCISE _____
_____
_____
_____

I PRACTICED...

- ☐ MEDITATION
- ☐ LOVING SELF-TALK
- ☐ DEEP BREATHING

RATE MY...

- ENERGY LEVEL ☆ ☆ ☆
- SELF-CARE ☆ ☆ ☆
- HUNGER/CRAVINGS ☆ ☆ ☆
- RELATIONSHIP WITH FOOD & EXERCISE ☆ ☆ ☆

ONE THING I WOULD LIKE TO KEEP WORKING ON _____
_____
_____

3 THINGS I AM GRATEFUL FOR TODAY

1. _____
2. _____
3. _____

# OF STEPS		% BODY FAT		WEIGHT	

saturday
WEEK 7

___/___/___

NUTRITION

	PROTEIN	STARCH	FRUIT	VEGETABLES	FATS
BREAKFAST 🕐					
MORNING SNACK 🕐					
LUNCH 🕐					
AFTERNOON SNACK 🕐					
DINNER 🕐					
EVENING SNACK 🕐					
TOTALS					

WATER 🍊 ② ③ ④ ⑤ ⑥ ⑦ ⑧ ⊕ ⊕ ⊕ ⊕

OTHER BEVERAGES _____

SUPPLEMENTS/MEDICATIONS _____

DIGESTION/BOWEL MOVEMENTS _____

> "GOOD THINGS ARE NOT DONE IN A HURRY."
> - GERMAN APHORISM

WHAT WOULD MAKE TODAY GREAT?

1. _____
2. _____
3. _____

MINDFULNESS

HOW DO I FEEL TODAY? _____

_____
_____
_____

MY MOOD IS...

- [ ] HAPPY
- [ ] FOCUSED
- [ ] ENERGETIC
- [ ] EXCITED
- [ ] SAD
- [ ] TIRED
- [ ] ANXIOUS
- [ ] ANGRY

FITNESS

EXERCISE _____
_____
_____
_____

I PRACTICED...

- [ ] MEDITATION
- [ ] LOVING SELF-TALK
- [ ] DEEP BREATHING

RATE MY...

- ENERGY LEVEL ☆ ☆ ☆
- SELF-CARE ☆ ☆ ☆
- HUNGER/CRAVINGS ☆ ☆ ☆
- RELATIONSHIP WITH FOOD & EXERCISE ☆ ☆ ☆

ONE THING I WOULD LIKE TO KEEP WORKING ON _____
_____
_____

3 THINGS I AM GRATEFUL FOR TODAY

1. _____
2. _____
3. _____

# OF STEPS		% BODY FAT		WEIGHT	

Sunday

WEEK 7

___/___/___

NUTRITION

	PROTEIN	STARCH	FRUIT	VEGETABLES	FATS
BREAKFAST 🕐					
MORNING SNACK 🕐					
LUNCH 🕐					
AFTERNOON SNACK 🕐					
DINNER 🕐					
EVENING SNACK 🕐					
TOTALS					

WATER 🍊 ② ③ ④ ⑤ ⑥ ⑦ ⑧ ⊕ ⊕ ⊕ ⊕

OTHER BEVERAGES _____

SUPPLEMENTS/MEDICATIONS _____

DIGESTION/BOWEL MOVEMENTS _____

**ASK YOURSELF TODAY:
HOW CAN I SNEAK EXTRA MOVEMENT
INTO MY WEEK?**

WHAT WOULD MAKE TODAY GREAT?

1. _____
2. _____
3. _____

MINDFULNESS

HOW DO I FEEL TODAY? _____

_____
_____
_____

MY MOOD IS...

- ☐ HAPPY
- ☐ FOCUSED
- ☐ ENERGETIC
- ☐ EXCITED
- ☐ SAD
- ☐ TIRED
- ☐ ANXIOUS
- ☐ ANGRY

FITNESS

EXERCISE _____

_____
_____
_____

I PRACTICED...

- ☐ MEDITATION
- ☐ LOVING SELF-TALK
- ☐ DEEP BREATHING

RATE MY...

- ENERGY LEVEL ☆ ☆ ☆
- SELF-CARE ☆ ☆ ☆
- HUNGER/CRAVINGS ☆ ☆ ☆
- RELATIONSHIP WITH FOOD & EXERCISE ☆ ☆ ☆

3 THINGS I AM GRATEFUL FOR TODAY

1. _____
2. _____
3. _____

ONE THING I WOULD LIKE TO KEEP WORKING ON _____

_____

# OF STEPS		% BODY FAT		WEIGHT	

I AM...

EMPOWERED

Week 8

Week 8 GOALS

GOALS FOR THIS WEEK

1) _____
2) _____
3) _____

EXERCISE PLAN

MONDAY _____
TUESDAY _____
WEDNESDAY _____
THURSDAY _____
FRIDAY _____
SATURDAY _____
SUNDAY _____

Week 8
MEAL PLAN & GROCERY LIST

MONDAY
- B
- L
- D

SNACKS

TUESDAY
- B
- L
- D

SNACKS

WEDNESDAY
- B
- L
- D

SNACKS

THURSDAY
- B
- L
- D

SNACKS

FRIDAY
- B
- L
- D

SNACKS

SATURDAY
- B
- L
- D

SNACKS

SUNDAY
- B
- L
- D

SNACKS

GROCERY LIST

Monday

WEEK 8 ___/___/___

NUTRITION

	PROTEIN	STARCH	FRUIT	VEGETABLES	FATS
BREAKFAST 🕐					
MORNING SNACK 🕐					
LUNCH 🕐					
AFTERNOON SNACK 🕐					
DINNER 🕐					
EVENING SNACK 🕐					
TOTALS					

WATER 💧 ② ③ ④ ⑤ ⑥ ⑦ ⑧ ⊕ ⊕ ⊕ ⊕

OTHER BEVERAGES _____

SUPPLEMENTS/MEDICATIONS _____

DIGESTION/BOWEL MOVEMENTS _____

"BY FAILING TO PREPARE YOU ARE PREPARING TO FAIL."
- BENJAMIN FRANKLIN

WHAT WOULD MAKE TODAY GREAT?

1. _____
2. _____
3. _____

MINDFULNESS

HOW DO I FEEL TODAY? _____
_____
_____
_____

MY MOOD IS...

- ☐ HAPPY
- ☐ FOCUSED
- ☐ ENERGETIC
- ☐ EXCITED
- ☐ SAD
- ☐ TIRED
- ☐ ANXIOUS
- ☐ ANGRY

FITNESS

EXERCISE _____
_____
_____
_____

I PRACTICED...

- ☐ MEDITATION
- ☐ LOVING SELF-TALK
- ☐ DEEP BREATHING

RATE MY...

- ENERGY LEVEL ☆ ☆ ☆
- SELF-CARE ☆ ☆ ☆
- HUNGER/CRAVINGS ☆ ☆ ☆
- RELATIONSHIP WITH FOOD & EXERCISE ☆ ☆ ☆

ONE THING I WOULD LIKE TO KEEP WORKING ON _____
_____
_____

3 THINGS I AM GRATEFUL FOR TODAY

1. _____
2. _____
3. _____

# OF STEPS		% BODY FAT		WEIGHT	

Tuesday
WEEK 8

___/___/___

NUTRITION

	PROTEIN	STARCH	FRUIT	VEGETABLES	FATS
BREAKFAST 🕐					
MORNING SNACK 🕐					
LUNCH 🕐					
AFTERNOON SNACK 🕐					
DINNER 🕐					
EVENING SNACK 🕐					
TOTALS					

WATER ① ② ③ ④ ⑤ ⑥ ⑦ ⑧ ⊕ ⊕ ⊕

OTHER BEVERAGES _____

SUPPLEMENTS/MEDICATIONS _____

DIGESTION/BOWEL MOVEMENTS _____

*"THE MIND IS EVERYTHING.
WHAT YOU THINK, YOU BECOME."
- GAUTAMA BUDDHA*

WHAT WOULD MAKE TODAY GREAT?

1. _____
2. _____
3. _____

MINDFULNESS

HOW DO I FEEL TODAY? _____
_____
_____
_____
_____

MY MOOD IS...

- ☐ HAPPY
- ☐ FOCUSED
- ☐ ENERGETIC
- ☐ EXCITED
- ☐ SAD
- ☐ TIRED
- ☐ ANXIOUS
- ☐ ANGRY

I PRACTICED...

- ☐ MEDITATION
- ☐ LOVING SELF-TALK
- ☐ DEEP BREATHING

FITNESS

EXERCISE _____
_____
_____
_____

RATE MY...

- ENERGY LEVEL ☆☆☆
- SELF-CARE ☆☆☆
- HUNGER/CRAVINGS ☆☆☆
- RELATIONSHIP WITH FOOD & EXERCISE ☆☆☆

ONE THING I WOULD LIKE TO KEEP WORKING ON _____
_____
_____

3 THINGS I AM GRATEFUL FOR TODAY

1. _____
2. _____
3. _____

| # OF STEPS | | % BODY FAT | | WEIGHT | |

Wednesday __/__/__
WEEK 8

NUTRITION

	PROTEIN	STARCH	FRUIT	VEGETABLES	FATS
BREAKFAST 🕐					
MORNING SNACK 🕐					
LUNCH 🕐					
AFTERNOON SNACK 🕐					
DINNER 🕐					
EVENING SNACK 🕐					
TOTALS					

WATER ⬥ ② ③ ④ ⑤ ⑥ ⑦ ⑧ ⊕ ⊕ ⊕ ⊕

OTHER BEVERAGES _____

SUPPLEMENTS/MEDICATIONS _____

DIGESTION/BOWEL MOVEMENTS _____

"FOREVER IS COMPOSED OF NOWS."
- EMILY DICKINSON

WHAT WOULD MAKE TODAY GREAT?

1. _____
2. _____
3. _____

MINDFULNESS

HOW DO I FEEL TODAY? _____

_____
_____
_____

MY MOOD IS...

- ☐ HAPPY   ☐ SAD
- ☐ FOCUSED   ☐ TIRED
- ☐ ENERGETIC   ☐ ANXIOUS
- ☐ EXCITED   ☐ ANGRY

I PRACTICED...

- ☐ MEDITATION
- ☐ LOVING SELF-TALK
- ☐ DEEP BREATHING

FITNESS

EXERCISE _____
_____
_____
_____

RATE MY...

- ENERGY LEVEL ☆☆☆
- SELF-CARE ☆☆☆
- HUNGER/CRAVINGS ☆☆☆
- RELATIONSHIP WITH FOOD & EXERCISE ☆☆☆

ONE THING I WOULD LIKE TO KEEP WORKING ON _____
_____
_____

3 THINGS I AM GRATEFUL FOR TODAY

1. _____
2. _____
3. _____

# OF STEPS		% BODY FAT		WEIGHT	

Thursday
WEEK 8

___/___/___

NUTRITION

	PROTEIN	STARCH	FRUIT	VEGETABLES	FATS
BREAKFAST 🕐					
MORNING SNACK 🕐					
LUNCH 🕐					
AFTERNOON SNACK 🕐					
DINNER 🕐					
EVENING SNACK 🕐					
TOTALS					

WATER 🍋 ② ③ ④ ⑤ ⑥ ⑦ ⑧ ⊕ ⊕ ⊕ ⊕

OTHER BEVERAGES _____

SUPPLEMENTS/MEDICATIONS _____

DIGESTION/BOWEL MOVEMENTS _____

"KNOW YOUR LIMITS BUT NEVER STOP TRYING TO EXCEED THEM."
— UNKNOWN

WHAT WOULD MAKE TODAY GREAT?

1. _____
2. _____
3. _____

MINDFULNESS

HOW DO I FEEL TODAY? _____
_____
_____
_____

MY MOOD IS...

- ☐ HAPPY
- ☐ FOCUSED
- ☐ ENERGETIC
- ☐ EXCITED
- ☐ SAD
- ☐ TIRED
- ☐ ANXIOUS
- ☐ ANGRY

FITNESS

EXERCISE _____
_____
_____
_____

I PRACTICED...

- ☐ MEDITATION
- ☐ LOVING SELF-TALK
- ☐ DEEP BREATHING

RATE MY...

- ENERGY LEVEL ☆☆☆
- SELF-CARE ☆☆☆
- HUNGER/CRAVINGS ☆☆☆
- RELATIONSHIP WITH FOOD & EXERCISE ☆☆☆

ONE THING I WOULD LIKE TO KEEP WORKING ON _____
_____
_____

3 THINGS I AM GRATEFUL FOR TODAY

1. _____
2. _____
3. _____

# OF STEPS	% BODY FAT	WEIGHT

Friday
WEEK 8

___/___/___

NUTRITION

	PROTEIN	STARCH	FRUIT	VEGETABLES	FATS
BREAKFAST 🕐					
MORNING SNACK 🕐					
LUNCH 🕐					
AFTERNOON SNACK 🕐					
DINNER 🕐					
EVENING SNACK 🕐					
TOTALS					

WATER 🍋 ② ③ ④ ⑤ ⑥ ⑦ ⑧ ➕ ➕ ➕ ➕

OTHER BEVERAGES _____

SUPPLEMENTS/MEDICATIONS _____

DIGESTION/BOWEL MOVEMENTS _____

"IT IS THE GREATEST OF ALL MISTAKES TO DO NOTHING BECAUSE YOU CAN ONLY DO A LITTLE."
- SYDNEY SMITH

WHAT WOULD MAKE TODAY GREAT?

1. _____
2. _____
3. _____

MINDFULNESS

HOW DO I FEEL TODAY? _____
_____
_____
_____

MY MOOD IS...
- ☐ HAPPY
- ☐ FOCUSED
- ☐ ENERGETIC
- ☐ EXCITED
- ☐ SAD
- ☐ TIRED
- ☐ ANXIOUS
- ☐ ANGRY

FITNESS

EXERCISE _____
_____
_____
_____

I PRACTICED...
- ☐ MEDITATION
- ☐ LOVING SELF-TALK
- ☐ DEEP BREATHING

RATE MY...

- ENERGY LEVEL ☆☆☆
- SELF-CARE ☆☆☆
- HUNGER/CRAVINGS ☆☆☆
- RELATIONSHIP WITH FOOD & EXERCISE ☆☆☆

ONE THING I WOULD LIKE TO KEEP WORKING ON _____
_____
_____

3 THINGS I AM GRATEFUL FOR TODAY

1. _____
2. _____
3. _____

☐ RECORD BODY MEASUREMENTS | # OF STEPS | % BODY FAT | WEIGHT

saturday
WEEK 8

___/___/___

NUTRITION

	PROTEIN	STARCH	FRUIT	VEGETABLES	FATS
BREAKFAST 🕐					
MORNING SNACK 🕐					
LUNCH 🕐					
AFTERNOON SNACK 🕐					
DINNER 🕐					
EVENING SNACK 🕐					
TOTALS					

WATER 💧 ② ③ ④ ⑤ ⑥ ⑦ ⑧ ➕ ➕ ➕ ➕

OTHER BEVERAGES _____

SUPPLEMENTS/MEDICATIONS _____

DIGESTION/BOWEL MOVEMENTS _____

> "THE BEST TEACHERS ARE THOSE WHO SHOW YOU WHERE TO LOOK, BUT DON'T TELL YOU WHAT TO SEE."
> - ALEXANDRA K. TRENFOR

WHAT WOULD MAKE TODAY GREAT?

1. _____
2. _____
3. _____

MINDFULNESS

HOW DO I FEEL TODAY? _____

_____
_____
_____

MY MOOD IS...

- ☐ HAPPY
- ☐ FOCUSED
- ☐ ENERGETIC
- ☐ EXCITED
- ☐ SAD
- ☐ TIRED
- ☐ ANXIOUS
- ☐ ANGRY

FITNESS

EXERCISE _____
_____
_____
_____

I PRACTICED...

- ☐ MEDITATION
- ☐ LOVING SELF-TALK
- ☐ DEEP BREATHING

RATE MY...

- ENERGY LEVEL ☆☆☆
- SELF-CARE ☆☆☆
- HUNGER/CRAVINGS ☆☆☆
- RELATIONSHIP WITH FOOD & EXERCISE ☆☆☆

ONE THING I WOULD LIKE TO KEEP WORKING ON _____
_____
_____

3 THINGS I AM GRATEFUL FOR TODAY

1. _____
2. _____
3. _____

# OF STEPS		% BODY FAT		WEIGHT	

Sunday
WEEK 8

___/___/___

NUTRITION

	PROTEIN	STARCH	FRUIT	VEGETABLES	FATS
BREAKFAST 🕐					
MORNING SNACK 🕐					
LUNCH 🕐					
AFTERNOON SNACK 🕐					
DINNER 🕐					
EVENING SNACK 🕐					
TOTALS					

WATER ① ② ③ ④ ⑤ ⑥ ⑦ ⑧ ⊕ ⊕ ⊕ ⊕

OTHER BEVERAGES _____

SUPPLEMENTS/MEDICATIONS _____

DIGESTION/BOWEL MOVEMENTS _____

**ASK YOURSELF TODAY:
HOW CAN I PUSH MYSELF PAST MY
COMFORT ZONE THIS WEEK?**

WHAT WOULD MAKE TODAY GREAT?

1. _____
2. _____
3. _____

MINDFULNESS

HOW DO I FEEL TODAY? _____

_____
_____
_____

MY MOOD IS...

- ☐ HAPPY
- ☐ SAD
- ☐ FOCUSED
- ☐ TIRED
- ☐ ENERGETIC
- ☐ ANXIOUS
- ☐ EXCITED
- ☐ ANGRY

FITNESS

EXERCISE _____
_____
_____

I PRACTICED...

- ☐ MEDITATION
- ☐ LOVING SELF-TALK
- ☐ DEEP BREATHING

RATE MY...

- ENERGY LEVEL ☆☆☆
- SELF-CARE ☆☆☆
- HUNGER/CRAVINGS ☆☆☆
- RELATIONSHIP WITH FOOD & EXERCISE ☆☆☆

3 THINGS I AM GRATEFUL FOR TODAY

1. _____
2. _____
3. _____

ONE THING I WOULD LIKE TO KEEP WORKING ON _____
_____
_____

# OF STEPS		% BODY FAT		WEIGHT	

I AM...

ABUNDANT

Week 9

Week 9 GOALS

GOALS FOR THIS WEEK

1

2

3

EXERCISE PLAN

MONDAY
TUESDAY
WEDNESDAY
THURSDAY
FRIDAY
SATURDAY
SUNDAY

Week 9
MEAL PLAN & GROCERY LIST

MONDAY
- B
- L
- D
- SNACKS

TUESDAY
- B
- L
- D
- SNACKS

WEDNESDAY
- B
- L
- D
- SNACKS

THURSDAY
- B
- L
- D
- SNACKS

FRIDAY
- B
- L
- D
- SNACKS

SATURDAY
- B
- L
- D
- SNACKS

SUNDAY
- B
- L
- D
- SNACKS

GROCERY LIST

Monday
WEEK 9

___/___/___

NUTRITION

		PROTEIN	STARCH	FRUIT	VEGETABLES	FATS
BREAKFAST 🕐						
MORNING SNACK 🕐						
LUNCH 🕐						
AFTERNOON SNACK 🕐						
DINNER 🕐						
EVENING SNACK 🕐						
TOTALS						

WATER 💧 ② ③ ④ ⑤ ⑥ ⑦ ⑧ ➕ ➕ ➕ ➕

OTHER BEVERAGES _____

SUPPLEMENTS/MEDICATIONS _____

DIGESTION/BOWEL MOVEMENTS _____

"YOU HAVE POWER OVER YOUR MIND, NOT OUTSIDE EVENTS. REALIZE THIS, AND YOU WILL FIND STRENGTH."
- MARCUS AURELIUS

WHAT WOULD MAKE TODAY GREAT?

1. _____
2. _____
3. _____

MINDFULNESS

HOW DO I FEEL TODAY? _____
_____
_____
_____

MY MOOD IS...

- ☐ HAPPY
- ☐ FOCUSED
- ☐ ENERGETIC
- ☐ EXCITED
- ☐ SAD
- ☐ TIRED
- ☐ ANXIOUS
- ☐ ANGRY

I PRACTICED...

- ☐ MEDITATION
- ☐ LOVING SELF-TALK
- ☐ DEEP BREATHING

FITNESS

EXERCISE _____
_____
_____
_____

RATE MY...

- ENERGY LEVEL ★ ★ ★
- SELF-CARE ★ ★ ★
- HUNGER/CRAVINGS ★ ★ ★
- RELATIONSHIP WITH FOOD & EXERCISE ★ ★ ★

ONE THING I WOULD LIKE TO KEEP WORKING ON _____
_____

3 THINGS I AM GRATEFUL FOR TODAY

1. _____
2. _____
3. _____

| # OF STEPS | | % BODY FAT | | WEIGHT | |

Tuesday
WEEK 9

___/___/___

NUTRITION

	PROTEIN	STARCH	FRUIT	VEGETABLES	FATS
BREAKFAST 🕐					
MORNING SNACK 🕐					
LUNCH 🕐					
AFTERNOON SNACK 🕐					
DINNER 🕐					
EVENING SNACK 🕐					
TOTALS					

WATER 🍊 2 3 4 5 6 7 8 ➕ ➕ ➕ ➕

OTHER BEVERAGES _____

SUPPLEMENTS/MEDICATIONS _____

DIGESTION/BOWEL MOVEMENTS _____

> "WHEN WORDS ARE BOTH TRUE AND KIND,
> THEY CAN CHANGE THE WORLD."
> - BUDDHA

WHAT WOULD MAKE TODAY GREAT?

1. _____
2. _____
3. _____

MINDFULNESS

HOW DO I FEEL TODAY? _____
_____
_____
_____

MY MOOD IS...

- ☐ HAPPY
- ☐ FOCUSED
- ☐ ENERGETIC
- ☐ EXCITED
- ☐ SAD
- ☐ TIRED
- ☐ ANXIOUS
- ☐ ANGRY

FITNESS

EXERCISE _____
_____
_____
_____

I PRACTICED...

- ☐ MEDITATION
- ☐ LOVING SELF-TALK
- ☐ DEEP BREATHING

RATE MY...

- ENERGY LEVEL ☆ ☆ ☆
- SELF-CARE ☆ ☆ ☆
- HUNGER/CRAVINGS ☆ ☆ ☆
- RELATIONSHIP WITH FOOD & EXERCISE ☆ ☆ ☆

ONE THING I WOULD LIKE TO KEEP WORKING ON _____
_____
_____

3 THINGS I AM GRATEFUL FOR TODAY

1. _____
2. _____
3. _____

| # OF STEPS | | % BODY FAT | | WEIGHT | |

Wednesday ___/___/___

WEEK 9

NUTRITION

		PROTEIN	STARCH	FRUIT	VEGETABLES	FATS
BREAKFAST 🕐						
MORNING SNACK 🕐						
LUNCH 🕐						
AFTERNOON SNACK 🕐						
DINNER 🕐						
EVENING SNACK 🕐						
TOTALS						

WATER 🍋 2 3 4 5 6 7 8 ➕ ➕ ➕ ➕

OTHER BEVERAGES _____

SUPPLEMENTS/MEDICATIONS _____

DIGESTION/BOWEL MOVEMENTS _____

> "LET'S NOT FORGET THAT THE LITTLE EMOTIONS ARE THE GREAT CAPTAINS OF OUR LIVES AND WE OBEY THEM WITHOUT REALIZING IT."
> — VINCENT VAN GOGH

WHAT WOULD MAKE TODAY GREAT?

1. _____
2. _____
3. _____

MINDFULNESS

HOW DO I FEEL TODAY? _____

_____
_____
_____

MY MOOD IS...

- ☐ HAPPY
- ☐ FOCUSED
- ☐ ENERGETIC
- ☐ EXCITED
- ☐ SAD
- ☐ TIRED
- ☐ ANXIOUS
- ☐ ANGRY

I PRACTICED...

- ☐ MEDITATION
- ☐ LOVING SELF-TALK
- ☐ DEEP BREATHING

FITNESS

EXERCISE _____

_____
_____
_____

RATE MY...

- ENERGY LEVEL ★★★
- SELF-CARE ★★★
- HUNGER/CRAVINGS ★★★
- RELATIONSHIP WITH FOOD & EXERCISE ★★★

ONE THING I WOULD LIKE TO KEEP WORKING ON _____

_____
_____

3 THINGS I AM GRATEFUL FOR TODAY

1. _____
2. _____
3. _____

# OF STEPS		% BODY FAT		WEIGHT	

Thursday
WEEK 9

___/___/___

NUTRITION

		PROTEIN	STARCH	FRUIT	VEGETABLES	FATS
BREAKFAST 🕐						
MORNING SNACK 🕐						
LUNCH 🕐						
AFTERNOON SNACK 🕐						
DINNER 🕐						
EVENING SNACK 🕐						
TOTALS						

WATER ◉ ② ③ ④ ⑤ ⑥ ⑦ ⑧ ⊕ ⊕ ⊕ ⊕

OTHER BEVERAGES _____

SUPPLEMENTS/MEDICATIONS _____

DIGESTION/BOWEL MOVEMENTS _____

> "NOTHING CAN STOP THE MAN WITH THE RIGHT MENTAL ATTITUDE FROM ACHIEVING HIS GOAL; NOTHING ON EARTH CAN HELP THE MAN WITH THE WRONG MENTAL ATTITUDE."
> - THOMAS JEFFERSON

WHAT WOULD MAKE TODAY GREAT?

1. _____
2. _____
3. _____

MINDFULNESS

HOW DO I FEEL TODAY? _____
_____
_____
_____

MY MOOD IS...

- ☐ HAPPY
- ☐ FOCUSED
- ☐ ENERGETIC
- ☐ EXCITED
- ☐ SAD
- ☐ TIRED
- ☐ ANXIOUS
- ☐ ANGRY

FITNESS

EXERCISE _____
_____
_____
_____

I PRACTICED...

- ☐ MEDITATION
- ☐ LOVING SELF-TALK
- ☐ DEEP BREATHING

RATE MY...

- ENERGY LEVEL ☆☆☆
- SELF-CARE ☆☆☆
- HUNGER/CRAVINGS ☆☆☆
- RELATIONSHIP WITH FOOD & EXERCISE ☆☆☆

ONE THING I WOULD LIKE TO KEEP WORKING ON _____
_____
_____

3 THINGS I AM GRATEFUL FOR TODAY

1. _____
2. _____
3. _____

# OF STEPS		% BODY FAT		WEIGHT	

Friday
WEEK 9

___/___/___

NUTRITION

	PROTEIN	STARCH	FRUIT	VEGETABLES	FATS
BREAKFAST 🕐					
MORNING SNACK 🕐					
LUNCH 🕐					
AFTERNOON SNACK 🕐					
DINNER 🕐					
EVENING SNACK 🕐					
TOTALS					

WATER 💧 2 3 4 5 6 7 8 ➕ ➕ ➕ ➕

OTHER BEVERAGES _____

SUPPLEMENTS/MEDICATIONS _____

DIGESTION/BOWEL MOVEMENTS _____

> "WHAT YOU THINK, YOU BECOME. WHAT YOU FEEL, YOU ATTRACT.
> WHAT YOU IMAGINE, YOU CREATE."
> - BUDDHA

WHAT WOULD MAKE TODAY GREAT?

1. _____
2. _____
3. _____

MINDFULNESS

HOW DO I FEEL TODAY? _____
_____
_____
_____

MY MOOD IS...

- ☐ HAPPY
- ☐ FOCUSED
- ☐ ENERGETIC
- ☐ EXCITED
- ☐ SAD
- ☐ TIRED
- ☐ ANXIOUS
- ☐ ANGRY

FITNESS

EXERCISE _____
_____
_____
_____

I PRACTICED...

- ☐ MEDITATION
- ☐ LOVING SELF-TALK
- ☐ DEEP BREATHING

RATE MY...

- ENERGY LEVEL ☆☆☆
- SELF-CARE ☆☆☆
- HUNGER/CRAVINGS ☆☆☆
- RELATIONSHIP WITH FOOD & EXERCISE ☆☆☆

ONE THING I WOULD LIKE TO KEEP WORKING ON _____
_____

3 THINGS I AM GRATEFUL FOR TODAY

1. _____
2. _____
3. _____

| # OF STEPS | | % BODY FAT | | WEIGHT | |

saturday
WEEK 9

___/___/___

NUTRITION

	PROTEIN	STARCH	FRUIT	VEGETABLES	FATS
BREAKFAST 🕐					
MORNING SNACK 🕐					
LUNCH 🕐					
AFTERNOON SNACK 🕐					
DINNER 🕐					
EVENING SNACK 🕐					
TOTALS					

WATER 🍊 ② ③ ④ ⑤ ⑥ ⑦ ⑧ ➕ ➕ ➕ ➕

OTHER BEVERAGES _____

SUPPLEMENTS/MEDICATIONS _____

DIGESTION/BOWEL MOVEMENTS _____

"DON'T FIND FAULT. FIND A REMEDY."
- HENRY FORD

WHAT WOULD MAKE TODAY GREAT?

1. _____
2. _____
3. _____

MINDFULNESS

HOW DO I FEEL TODAY? _____
_____
_____
_____

MY MOOD IS...

- ☐ HAPPY   ☐ SAD
- ☐ FOCUSED   ☐ TIRED
- ☐ ENERGETIC ☐ ANXIOUS
- ☐ EXCITED   ☐ ANGRY

FITNESS

EXERCISE _____
_____
_____
_____

I PRACTICED...

- ☐ MEDITATION
- ☐ LOVING SELF-TALK
- ☐ DEEP BREATHING

RATE MY...

- ENERGY LEVEL ☆ ☆ ☆
- SELF-CARE ☆ ☆ ☆
- HUNGER/CRAVINGS ☆ ☆ ☆
- RELATIONSHIP WITH FOOD & EXERCISE ☆ ☆ ☆

ONE THING I WOULD LIKE TO KEEP WORKING ON _____
_____
_____

3 THINGS I AM GRATEFUL FOR TODAY

1. _____
2. _____
3. _____

| # OF STEPS | | % BODY FAT | | WEIGHT | |

Sunday
WEEK 9

___/___/___

NUTRITION

		PROTEIN	STARCH	FRUIT	VEGETABLES	FATS
BREAKFAST 🕐						
MORNING SNACK 🕐						
LUNCH 🕐						
AFTERNOON SNACK 🕐						
DINNER 🕐						
EVENING SNACK 🕐						
TOTALS						

WATER 💧 ② ③ ④ ⑤ ⑥ ⑦ ⑧ ➕ ➕ ➕ ➕

OTHER BEVERAGES _____

SUPPLEMENTS/MEDICATIONS _____

DIGESTION/BOWEL MOVEMENTS _____

ASK YOURSELF TODAY:
WHAT LIMITING BELIEFS ABOUT MYSELF DO I HAVE?

WHAT WOULD MAKE TODAY GREAT?

1. _____
2. _____
3. _____

MINDFULNESS

HOW DO I FEEL TODAY? _____
_____
_____
_____

MY MOOD IS...

- ☐ HAPPY
- ☐ FOCUSED
- ☐ ENERGETIC
- ☐ EXCITED
- ☐ SAD
- ☐ TIRED
- ☐ ANXIOUS
- ☐ ANGRY

FITNESS

EXERCISE _____
_____
_____
_____

I PRACTICED...

- ☐ MEDITATION
- ☐ LOVING SELF-TALK
- ☐ DEEP BREATHING

RATE MY...

- ENERGY LEVEL ☆ ☆ ☆
- SELF-CARE ☆ ☆ ☆
- HUNGER/CRAVINGS ☆ ☆ ☆
- RELATIONSHIP WITH FOOD & EXERCISE ☆ ☆ ☆

ONE THING I WOULD LIKE TO KEEP WORKING ON _____
_____
_____

3 THINGS I AM GRATEFUL FOR TODAY

1. _____
2. _____
3. _____

# OF STEPS		% BODY FAT		WEIGHT	

I AM...

GROUNDED

Week 10

Week 10 GOALS

GOALS FOR THIS WEEK

1. _____
2. _____
3. _____

EXERCISE PLAN

MONDAY	_____
TUESDAY	_____
WEDNESDAY	_____
THURSDAY	_____
FRIDAY	_____
SATURDAY	_____
SUNDAY	_____

Week 10
MEAL PLAN & GROCERY LIST

MONDAY
- (B)
- (L)
- (D)

SNACKS

TUESDAY
- (B)
- (L)
- (D)

SNACKS

WEDNESDAY
- (B)
- (L)
- (D)

SNACKS

THURSDAY
- (B)
- (L)
- (D)

SNACKS

FRIDAY
- (B)
- (L)
- (D)

SNACKS

SATURDAY
- (B)
- (L)
- (D)

SNACKS

SUNDAY
- (B)
- (L)
- (D)

SNACKS

GROCERY LIST

Monday
WEEK 10

___/___/___

NUTRITION

	PROTEIN	STARCH	FRUIT	VEGETABLES	FATS
BREAKFAST 🕐					
MORNING SNACK 🕐					
LUNCH 🕐					
AFTERNOON SNACK 🕐					
DINNER 🕐					
EVENING SNACK 🕐					
TOTALS					

WATER ① ② ③ ④ ⑤ ⑥ ⑦ ⑧ ⊕ ⊕ ⊕

OTHER BEVERAGES _____

SUPPLEMENTS/MEDICATIONS _____

DIGESTION/BOWEL MOVEMENTS _____

"DEAL WITH THE BIG WHILE IT'S STILL SMALL."
- LAO TZU

WHAT WOULD MAKE TODAY GREAT?

1. _____
2. _____
3. _____

MINDFULNESS

HOW DO I FEEL TODAY? _____
_____
_____
_____

MY MOOD IS...

- ☐ HAPPY
- ☐ FOCUSED
- ☐ ENERGETIC
- ☐ EXCITED
- ☐ SAD
- ☐ TIRED
- ☐ ANXIOUS
- ☐ ANGRY

I PRACTICED...

- ☐ MEDITATION
- ☐ LOVING SELF-TALK
- ☐ DEEP BREATHING

FITNESS

EXERCISE _____
_____
_____
_____

RATE MY...

- ENERGY LEVEL ☆☆☆
- SELF-CARE ☆☆☆
- HUNGER/CRAVINGS ☆☆☆
- RELATIONSHIP WITH FOOD & EXERCISE ☆☆☆

ONE THING I WOULD LIKE TO KEEP WORKING ON _____
_____
_____

3 THINGS I AM GRATEFUL FOR TODAY

1. _____
2. _____
3. _____

# OF STEPS	% BODY FAT	WEIGHT

Tuesday
WEEK 10

___/___/___

NUTRITION

		PROTEIN	STARCH	FRUIT	VEGETABLES	FATS
BREAKFAST 🕐						
MORNING SNACK 🕐						
LUNCH 🕐						
AFTERNOON SNACK 🕐						
DINNER 🕐						
EVENING SNACK 🕐						
TOTALS						

WATER 💧 ② ③ ④ ⑤ ⑥ ⑦ ⑧ ⊕ ⊕ ⊕ ⊕

OTHER BEVERAGES _____

SUPPLEMENTS/MEDICATIONS _____

DIGESTION/BOWEL MOVEMENTS _____

> "THE DIFFICULTY LIES NOT SO MUCH IN DEVELOPING NEW IDEAS AS IN ESCAPING FROM OLD ONES."
> - JOHN MAYNARD KEYES

WHAT WOULD MAKE TODAY GREAT?

1. _____
2. _____
3. _____

MINDFULNESS

HOW DO I FEEL TODAY? _____

_____
_____
_____

MY MOOD IS...

- ☐ HAPPY
- ☐ FOCUSED
- ☐ ENERGETIC
- ☐ EXCITED
- ☐ SAD
- ☐ TIRED
- ☐ ANXIOUS
- ☐ ANGRY

I PRACTICED...

- ☐ MEDITATION
- ☐ LOVING SELF-TALK
- ☐ DEEP BREATHING

FITNESS

EXERCISE _____

_____
_____
_____

RATE MY...

- ENERGY LEVEL ☆☆☆
- SELF-CARE ☆☆☆
- HUNGER/CRAVINGS ☆☆☆
- RELATIONSHIP WITH FOOD & EXERCISE ☆☆☆

ONE THING I WOULD LIKE TO KEEP WORKING ON _____

_____
_____

3 THINGS I AM GRATEFUL FOR TODAY

1. _____
2. _____
3. _____

# OF STEPS	% BODY FAT	WEIGHT

Wednesday ___/___/___
WEEK 10

NUTRITION

	PROTEIN	STARCH	FRUIT	VEGETABLES	FATS
BREAKFAST 🕐					
MORNING SNACK 🕐					
LUNCH 🕐					
AFTERNOON SNACK 🕐					
DINNER 🕐					
EVENING SNACK 🕐					
TOTALS					

WATER 💧 ② ③ ④ ⑤ ⑥ ⑦ ⑧ ⊕ ⊕ ⊕ ⊕

OTHER BEVERAGES _____

SUPPLEMENTS/MEDICATIONS _____

DIGESTION/BOWEL MOVEMENTS _____

"ANY TIME YOU FIND YOURSELF FEELING SO SURE ABOUT ANYTHING, IT MIGHT BE TIME TO QUESTION IT."
— JENNIFER ANTHONY

WHAT WOULD MAKE TODAY GREAT?

1. _____
2. _____
3. _____

MINDFULNESS

HOW DO I FEEL TODAY? _____
_____
_____
_____

MY MOOD IS...
- ☐ HAPPY
- ☐ FOCUSED
- ☐ ENERGETIC
- ☐ EXCITED
- ☐ SAD
- ☐ TIRED
- ☐ ANXIOUS
- ☐ ANGRY

I PRACTICED...
- ☐ MEDITATION
- ☐ LOVING SELF-TALK
- ☐ DEEP BREATHING

FITNESS

EXERCISE _____
_____
_____
_____

RATE MY...
- ENERGY LEVEL ☆☆☆
- SELF-CARE ☆☆☆
- HUNGER/CRAVINGS ☆☆☆
- RELATIONSHIP WITH FOOD & EXERCISE ☆☆☆

ONE THING I WOULD LIKE TO KEEP WORKING ON _____
_____
_____

3 THINGS I AM GRATEFUL FOR TODAY

1. _____
2. _____
3. _____

# OF STEPS		% BODY FAT		WEIGHT	

Thursday

WEEK 10 ___/___/___

NUTRITION

		PROTEIN	STARCH	FRUIT	VEGETABLES	FATS
BREAKFAST 🕐						
MORNING SNACK 🕐						
LUNCH 🕐						
AFTERNOON SNACK 🕐						
DINNER 🕐						
EVENING SNACK 🕐						
TOTALS						

WATER 💧 ② ③ ④ ⑤ ⑥ ⑦ ⑧ ⊕ ⊕ ⊕ ⊕

OTHER BEVERAGES _____

SUPPLEMENTS/MEDICATIONS _____

DIGESTION/BOWEL MOVEMENTS _____

> "EXPERIENCE IS THE TEACHER OF ALL THINGS."
> - JULIUS CAESAR

WHAT WOULD MAKE TODAY GREAT?

1. _____
2. _____
3. _____

MINDFULNESS

HOW DO I FEEL TODAY? _____
_____
_____
_____

MY MOOD IS...

- ☐ HAPPY
- ☐ FOCUSED
- ☐ ENERGETIC
- ☐ EXCITED
- ☐ SAD
- ☐ TIRED
- ☐ ANXIOUS
- ☐ ANGRY

I PRACTICED...

- ☐ MEDITATION
- ☐ LOVING SELF-TALK
- ☐ DEEP BREATHING

FITNESS

EXERCISE _____
_____
_____
_____

RATE MY...

- ENERGY LEVEL ☆☆☆
- SELF-CARE ☆☆☆
- HUNGER/CRAVINGS ☆☆☆
- RELATIONSHIP WITH FOOD & EXERCISE ☆☆☆

ONE THING I WOULD LIKE TO KEEP WORKING ON _____
_____
_____

3 THINGS I AM GRATEFUL FOR TODAY

1. _____
2. _____
3. _____

| # OF STEPS | | % BODY FAT | | WEIGHT | |

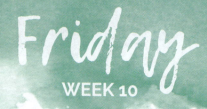

Friday
WEEK 10

___/___/___

NUTRITION

	PROTEIN	STARCH	FRUIT	VEGETABLES	FATS
BREAKFAST 🕐					
MORNING SNACK 🕐					
LUNCH 🕐					
AFTERNOON SNACK 🕐					
DINNER 🕐					
EVENING SNACK 🕐					
TOTALS					

WATER 💧 ② ③ ④ ⑤ ⑥ ⑦ ⑧ ➕ ➕ ➕

OTHER BEVERAGES _____

SUPPLEMENTS/MEDICATIONS _____

DIGESTION/BOWEL MOVEMENTS _____

> "THE TREES THAT ARE SLOW TO GROW BEAR
> THE BEST FRUIT."
> - MOLIERE

WHAT WOULD MAKE TODAY GREAT?

1. _____
2. _____
3. _____

MINDFULNESS

HOW DO I FEEL TODAY? _____

_____
_____
_____

MY MOOD IS...

- [ ] HAPPY
- [ ] FOCUSED
- [ ] ENERGETIC
- [ ] EXCITED
- [ ] SAD
- [ ] TIRED
- [ ] ANXIOUS
- [ ] ANGRY

FITNESS

EXERCISE _____
_____
_____
_____

I PRACTICED...

- [ ] MEDITATION
- [ ] LOVING SELF-TALK
- [ ] DEEP BREATHING

RATE MY...

ENERGY LEVEL ☆ ☆ ☆
SELF-CARE ☆ ☆ ☆
HUNGER/CRAVINGS ☆ ☆ ☆
RELATIONSHIP WITH FOOD & EXERCISE ☆ ☆ ☆

ONE THING I WOULD LIKE TO KEEP WORKING ON _____
_____

3 THINGS I AM GRATEFUL FOR TODAY

1. _____
2. _____
3. _____

- [ ] RECORD BODY MEASUREMENTS | # OF STEPS ___ | % BODY FAT ___ | WEIGHT ___

saturday ___/___/___
WEEK 10

NUTRITION

	PROTEIN	STARCH	FRUIT	VEGETABLES	FATS
BREAKFAST 🕐					
MORNING SNACK 🕐					
LUNCH 🕐					
AFTERNOON SNACK 🕐					
DINNER 🕐					
EVENING SNACK 🕐					
TOTALS					

WATER ◈ ② ③ ④ ⑤ ⑥ ⑦ ⑧ ⊕ ⊕ ⊕ ⊕

OTHER BEVERAGES _____

SUPPLEMENTS/MEDICATIONS _____

DIGESTION/BOWEL MOVEMENTS _____

> "THE RIGHT AND WRONG ANSWERS SHOULD
> COME FROM YOUR HEART."
> - UNKNOWN

WHAT WOULD MAKE TODAY GREAT?

1. _____
2. _____
3. _____

MINDFULNESS

HOW DO I FEEL TODAY? _____
_____
_____
_____

MY MOOD IS...

- ☐ HAPPY
- ☐ FOCUSED
- ☐ ENERGETIC
- ☐ EXCITED
- ☐ SAD
- ☐ TIRED
- ☐ ANXIOUS
- ☐ ANGRY

FITNESS

EXERCISE _____
_____
_____
_____

I PRACTICED...

- ☐ MEDITATION
- ☐ LOVING SELF-TALK
- ☐ DEEP BREATHING

RATE MY...

- ENERGY LEVEL ☆☆☆
- SELF-CARE ☆☆☆
- HUNGER/CRAVINGS ☆☆☆
- RELATIONSHIP WITH FOOD & EXERCISE ☆☆☆

ONE THING I WOULD LIKE TO KEEP WORKING ON _____
_____
_____

3 THINGS I AM GRATEFUL FOR TODAY

1. _____
2. _____
3. _____

# OF STEPS	% BODY FAT	WEIGHT

Sunday
WEEK 10

___/___/___

NUTRITION

	PROTEIN	STARCH	FRUIT	VEGETABLES	FATS
BREAKFAST 🕐					
MORNING SNACK 🕐					
LUNCH 🕐					
AFTERNOON SNACK 🕐					
DINNER 🕐					
EVENING SNACK 🕐					
TOTALS					

WATER 🍊 ② ③ ④ ⑤ ⑥ ⑦ ⑧ ⊕ ⊕ ⊕ ⊕

OTHER BEVERAGES _____

SUPPLEMENTS/MEDICATIONS _____

DIGESTION/BOWEL MOVEMENTS _____

**ASK YOURSELF TODAY:
WHAT DO I NEED TO LET GO OF TO MOVE
FORWARD IN MY LIFE?**

WHAT WOULD MAKE TODAY GREAT?

1. _____
2. _____
3. _____

MINDFULNESS

HOW DO I FEEL TODAY? _____
_____
_____
_____

MY MOOD IS...

- ☐ HAPPY
- ☐ FOCUSED
- ☐ ENERGETIC
- ☐ EXCITED
- ☐ SAD
- ☐ TIRED
- ☐ ANXIOUS
- ☐ ANGRY

FITNESS

EXERCISE _____
_____
_____
_____

I PRACTICED...

- ☐ MEDITATION
- ☐ LOVING SELF-TALK
- ☐ DEEP BREATHING

RATE MY...

- ENERGY LEVEL ☆ ☆ ☆
- SELF-CARE ☆ ☆ ☆
- HUNGER/CRAVINGS ☆ ☆ ☆
- RELATIONSHIP WITH FOOD & EXERCISE ☆ ☆ ☆

ONE THING I WOULD LIKE TO KEEP WORKING ON _____
_____
_____

3 THINGS I AM GRATEFUL FOR TODAY

1. _____
2. _____
3. _____

| # OF STEPS | | % BODY FAT | | WEIGHT | |

I AM...
HEALTHY

Week 11

Week 11 GOALS

GOALS FOR THIS WEEK

1. _____

2. _____

3. _____

EXERCISE PLAN

MONDAY _____
TUESDAY _____
WEDNESDAY _____
THURSDAY _____
FRIDAY _____
SATURDAY _____
SUNDAY _____

Week 11
MEAL PLAN & GROCERY LIST

MONDAY
- B
- L
- D

SNACKS

TUESDAY
- B
- L
- D

SNACKS

WEDNESDAY
- B
- L
- D

SNACKS

THURSDAY
- B
- L
- D

SNACKS

FRIDAY
- B
- L
- D

SNACKS

SATURDAY
- B
- L
- D

SNACKS

SUNDAY
- B
- L
- D

SNACKS

GROCERY LIST

Monday

WEEK 11

___/___/___

NUTRITION

		PROTEIN	STARCH	FRUIT	VEGETABLES	FATS
BREAKFAST 🕐						
MORNING SNACK 🕐						
LUNCH 🕐						
AFTERNOON SNACK 🕐						
DINNER 🕐						
EVENING SNACK 🕐						
TOTALS						

WATER 🍊 2 3 4 5 6 7 8 ⊕ ⊕ ⊕ ⊕

OTHER BEVERAGES _____

SUPPLEMENTS/MEDICATIONS _____

DIGESTION/BOWEL MOVEMENTS _____

"WHAT YOU SEEK IS SEEKING YOU."
- RUMI

WHAT WOULD MAKE TODAY GREAT?

1. _____
2. _____
3. _____

MINDFULNESS

HOW DO I FEEL TODAY? _____

_____
_____
_____

MY MOOD IS...

- ☐ HAPPY
- ☐ FOCUSED
- ☐ ENERGETIC
- ☐ EXCITED
- ☐ SAD
- ☐ TIRED
- ☐ ANXIOUS
- ☐ ANGRY

FITNESS

EXERCISE _____

_____
_____
_____

I PRACTICED...

- ☐ MEDITATION
- ☐ LOVING SELF-TALK
- ☐ DEEP BREATHING

RATE MY...

- ENERGY LEVEL ☆ ☆ ☆
- SELF-CARE ☆ ☆ ☆
- HUNGER/CRAVINGS ☆ ☆ ☆
- RELATIONSHIP WITH FOOD & EXERCISE ☆ ☆ ☆

ONE THING I WOULD LIKE TO KEEP WORKING ON _____

_____
_____

3 THINGS I AM GRATEFUL FOR TODAY

1. _____
2. _____
3. _____

# OF STEPS	% BODY FAT	WEIGHT

Tuesday
WEEK 11

___/___/___

NUTRITION

	PROTEIN	STARCH	FRUIT	VEGETABLES	FATS
BREAKFAST					
MORNING SNACK					
LUNCH					
AFTERNOON SNACK					
DINNER					
EVENING SNACK					
TOTALS					

WATER 🍊 ② ③ ④ ⑤ ⑥ ⑦ ⑧ ⊕ ⊕ ⊕ ⊕

OTHER BEVERAGES _____

SUPPLEMENTS/MEDICATIONS _____

DIGESTION/BOWEL MOVEMENTS _____

> "I AM OUT WITH LANTERNS LOOKING FOR MYSELF."
> - EMILY DICKINSON

WHAT WOULD MAKE TODAY GREAT?

1. _____
2. _____
3. _____

MINDFULNESS

HOW DO I FEEL TODAY? _____

_____
_____
_____

MY MOOD IS...

- ☐ HAPPY
- ☐ FOCUSED
- ☐ ENERGETIC
- ☐ EXCITED
- ☐ SAD
- ☐ TIRED
- ☐ ANXIOUS
- ☐ ANGRY

FITNESS

EXERCISE _____
_____
_____
_____

I PRACTICED...

- ☐ MEDITATION
- ☐ LOVING SELF-TALK
- ☐ DEEP BREATHING

RATE MY...

- ENERGY LEVEL ☆ ☆ ☆
- SELF-CARE ☆ ☆ ☆
- HUNGER/CRAVINGS ☆ ☆ ☆
- RELATIONSHIP WITH FOOD & EXERCISE ☆ ☆ ☆

ONE THING I WOULD LIKE TO KEEP WORKING ON _____
_____
_____

3 THINGS I AM GRATEFUL FOR TODAY

1. _____
2. _____
3. _____

| # OF STEPS | | % BODY FAT | | WEIGHT | |

Wednesday ___/___/___

WEEK 11

NUTRITION

	PROTEIN	STARCH	FRUIT	VEGETABLES	FATS
BREAKFAST 🕐					
MORNING SNACK 🕐					
LUNCH 🕐					
AFTERNOON SNACK 🕐					
DINNER 🕐					
EVENING SNACK 🕐					
TOTALS					

WATER 🍊 ② ③ ④ ⑤ ⑥ ⑦ ⑧ ⊕ ⊕ ⊕

OTHER BEVERAGES _____

SUPPLEMENTS/MEDICATIONS _____

DIGESTION/BOWEL MOVEMENTS _____

> "THE MIND, ONCE STRETCHED BY A NEW IDEA,
> NEVER REGAINS ITS ORIGINAL DIMENSIONS."
> - OLIVER WENDELL HOLMES

WHAT WOULD MAKE TODAY GREAT?

1) _____
2) _____
3) _____

MINDFULNESS

HOW DO I FEEL TODAY? _____
_____
_____
_____

MY MOOD IS...

- ☐ HAPPY
- ☐ FOCUSED
- ☐ ENERGETIC
- ☐ EXCITED
- ☐ SAD
- ☐ TIRED
- ☐ ANXIOUS
- ☐ ANGRY

FITNESS

EXERCISE _____
_____
_____
_____

I PRACTICED...

- ☐ MEDITATION
- ☐ LOVING SELF-TALK
- ☐ DEEP BREATHING

RATE MY...

- ENERGY LEVEL ☆ ☆ ☆
- SELF-CARE ☆ ☆ ☆
- HUNGER/CRAVINGS ☆ ☆ ☆
- RELATIONSHIP WITH FOOD & EXERCISE ☆ ☆ ☆

ONE THING I WOULD LIKE TO KEEP WORKING ON _____
_____
_____

3 THINGS I AM GRATEFUL FOR TODAY

1) _____
2) _____
3) _____

| # OF STEPS | | % BODY FAT | | WEIGHT | |

Thursday ___/___/___
WEEK 11

NUTRITION

	PROTEIN	STARCH	FRUIT	VEGETABLES	FATS
BREAKFAST 🕐					
MORNING SNACK 🕐					
LUNCH 🕐					
AFTERNOON SNACK 🕐					
DINNER 🕐					
EVENING SNACK 🕐					
TOTALS					

WATER 💧 ② ③ ④ ⑤ ⑥ ⑦ ⑧ ➕ ➕ ➕ ➕

OTHER BEVERAGES _____

SUPPLEMENTS/MEDICATIONS _____

DIGESTION/BOWEL MOVEMENTS _____

> "DO NOT DWELL IN THE PAST, DO NOT DREAM OF THE FUTURE,
> CONCENTRATE THE MIND ON THE PRESENT MOMENT."
> - GAUTAMA BUDDHA

WHAT WOULD MAKE TODAY GREAT?

1. _____
2. _____
3. _____

MINDFULNESS

HOW DO I FEEL TODAY? _____
_____
_____
_____

MY MOOD IS...

- ☐ HAPPY
- ☐ FOCUSED
- ☐ ENERGETIC
- ☐ EXCITED
- ☐ SAD
- ☐ TIRED
- ☐ ANXIOUS
- ☐ ANGRY

FITNESS

EXERCISE _____
_____
_____
_____

I PRACTICED...

- ☐ MEDITATION
- ☐ LOVING SELF-TALK
- ☐ DEEP BREATHING

RATE MY...

- ENERGY LEVEL ☆ ☆ ☆
- SELF-CARE ☆ ☆ ☆
- HUNGER/CRAVINGS ☆ ☆ ☆
- RELATIONSHIP WITH FOOD & EXERCISE ☆ ☆ ☆

ONE THING I WOULD LIKE TO KEEP WORKING ON _____
_____
_____

3 THINGS I AM GRATEFUL FOR TODAY

1. _____
2. _____
3. _____

# OF STEPS		% BODY FAT		WEIGHT	

Friday

WEEK 11

___/___/___

NUTRITION

	PROTEIN	STARCH	FRUIT	VEGETABLES	FATS
BREAKFAST					
MORNING SNACK					
LUNCH					
AFTERNOON SNACK					
DINNER					
EVENING SNACK					
TOTALS					

WATER 2 3 4 5 6 7 8 + + + +

OTHER BEVERAGES _____

SUPPLEMENTS/MEDICATIONS _____

DIGESTION/BOWEL MOVEMENTS _____

> "FOR SUCCESS, ATTITUDE IS EQUALLY AS IMPORTANT AS ABILITY."
> - WALTER SCOTT

WHAT WOULD MAKE TODAY GREAT?

1. _____
2. _____
3. _____

MINDFULNESS

HOW DO I FEEL TODAY? _____

_____
_____
_____

MY MOOD IS...

- [ ] HAPPY
- [ ] FOCUSED
- [ ] ENERGETIC
- [ ] EXCITED
- [ ] SAD
- [ ] TIRED
- [ ] ANXIOUS
- [ ] ANGRY

FITNESS

EXERCISE _____
_____
_____
_____

RATE MY...

- ENERGY LEVEL ☆☆☆
- SELF-CARE ☆☆☆
- HUNGER/CRAVINGS ☆☆☆
- RELATIONSHIP WITH FOOD & EXERCISE ☆☆☆

ONE THING I WOULD LIKE TO KEEP WORKING ON _____
_____
_____

I PRACTICED...

- [ ] MEDITATION
- [ ] LOVING SELF-TALK
- [ ] DEEP BREATHING

3 THINGS I AM GRATEFUL FOR TODAY

1. _____
2. _____
3. _____

# OF STEPS		% BODY FAT		WEIGHT	

saturday
WEEK 11

___/___/___

NUTRITION

		PROTEIN	STARCH	FRUIT	VEGETABLES	FATS
BREAKFAST 🕐						
MORNING SNACK 🕐						
LUNCH 🕐						
AFTERNOON SNACK 🕐						
DINNER 🕐						
EVENING SNACK 🕐						
TOTALS						

WATER ◊ ② ③ ④ ⑤ ⑥ ⑦ ⑧ ⊕ ⊕ ⊕ ⊕

OTHER BEVERAGES _____

SUPPLEMENTS/MEDICATIONS _____

DIGESTION/BOWEL MOVEMENTS _____

> "TRUE HAPPINESS IS... TO ENJOY THE PRESENT, WITHOUT ANXIOUS DEPENDENCE UPON THE FUTURE."
> - LUCIUS ANNAEUS SENECA

WHAT WOULD MAKE TODAY GREAT?

1. _____
2. _____
3. _____

MINDFULNESS

HOW DO I FEEL TODAY? _____

_____

_____

MY MOOD IS...

- ☐ HAPPY
- ☐ FOCUSED
- ☐ ENERGETIC
- ☐ EXCITED
- ☐ SAD
- ☐ TIRED
- ☐ ANXIOUS
- ☐ ANGRY

FITNESS

EXERCISE _____

_____

_____

_____

I PRACTICED...

- ☐ MEDITATION
- ☐ LOVING SELF-TALK
- ☐ DEEP BREATHING

RATE MY...

- ENERGY LEVEL ☆ ☆ ☆
- SELF-CARE ☆ ☆ ☆
- HUNGER/CRAVINGS ☆ ☆ ☆
- RELATIONSHIP WITH FOOD & EXERCISE ☆ ☆ ☆

ONE THING I WOULD LIKE TO KEEP WORKING ON _____

_____

_____

3 THINGS I AM GRATEFUL FOR TODAY

1. _____
2. _____
3. _____

# OF STEPS		% BODY FAT		WEIGHT	

Sunday
WEEK 11

___/___/___

NUTRITION

	PROTEIN	STARCH	FRUIT	VEGETABLES	FATS
BREAKFAST 🕐					
MORNING SNACK 🕐					
LUNCH 🕐					
AFTERNOON SNACK 🕐					
DINNER 🕐					
EVENING SNACK 🕐					
TOTALS					

WATER 🍊 ② ③ ④ ⑤ ⑥ ⑦ ⑧ ⊕ ⊕ ⊕ ⊕

OTHER BEVERAGES _____

SUPPLEMENTS/MEDICATIONS _____

DIGESTION/BOWEL MOVEMENTS _____

**ASK YOURSELF TODAY:
WHAT ARE MY PERSONALITY STRENGTHS?**

WHAT WOULD MAKE TODAY GREAT?

1. _____
2. _____
3. _____

MINDFULNESS

HOW DO I FEEL TODAY? _____
_____
_____
_____

MY MOOD IS...

- ☐ HAPPY
- ☐ FOCUSED
- ☐ ENERGETIC
- ☐ EXCITED
- ☐ SAD
- ☐ TIRED
- ☐ ANXIOUS
- ☐ ANGRY

FITNESS

EXERCISE _____
_____
_____

I PRACTICED...

- ☐ MEDITATION
- ☐ LOVING SELF-TALK
- ☐ DEEP BREATHING

RATE MY...

- ENERGY LEVEL ☆ ☆ ☆
- SELF-CARE ☆ ☆ ☆
- HUNGER/CRAVINGS ☆ ☆ ☆
- RELATIONSHIP WITH FOOD & EXERCISE ☆ ☆ ☆

ONE THING I WOULD LIKE TO KEEP WORKING ON _____
_____
_____

3 THINGS I AM GRATEFUL FOR TODAY

1. _____
2. _____
3. _____

# OF STEPS	% BODY FAT	WEIGHT

I AM...

GRATEFUL

Week 12

Week 12 GOALS

GOALS FOR THIS WEEK

1. _____
   _____
   _____

2. _____
   _____
   _____

3. _____
   _____
   _____

EXERCISE PLAN

MONDAY	_____
TUESDAY	_____
WEDNESDAY	_____
THURSDAY	_____
FRIDAY	_____
SATURDAY	_____
SUNDAY	_____

Week 12
MEAL PLAN & GROCERY LIST

MONDAY
- B
- L
- D

SNACKS

TUESDAY
- B
- L
- D

SNACKS

WEDNESDAY
- B
- L
- D

SNACKS

THURSDAY
- B
- L
- D

SNACKS

FRIDAY
- B
- L
- D

SNACKS

SATURDAY
- B
- L
- D

SNACKS

SUNDAY
- B
- L
- D

SNACKS

GROCERY LIST

Monday
WEEK 12

___/___/___

NUTRITION

	PROTEIN	STARCH	FRUIT	VEGETABLES	FATS
BREAKFAST 🕐					
MORNING SNACK 🕐					
LUNCH 🕐					
AFTERNOON SNACK 🕐					
DINNER 🕐					
EVENING SNACK 🕐					
TOTALS					

WATER 🍋 2 3 4 5 6 7 8 ⊕ ⊕ ⊕ ⊕

OTHER BEVERAGES _____

SUPPLEMENTS/MEDICATIONS _____

DIGESTION/BOWEL MOVEMENTS _____

*"THAT WHICH IS FALSE TROUBLES THE HEART,
BUT TRUTH BRINGS JOYOUS TRANQUILITY."
- RUMI*

WHAT WOULD MAKE TODAY GREAT?

1. _____
2. _____
3. _____

MINDFULNESS

HOW DO I FEEL TODAY? _____

_____
_____
_____

MY MOOD IS...

- ☐ HAPPY
- ☐ FOCUSED
- ☐ ENERGETIC
- ☐ EXCITED
- ☐ SAD
- ☐ TIRED
- ☐ ANXIOUS
- ☐ ANGRY

FITNESS

EXERCISE _____

_____
_____
_____

I PRACTICED...

- ☐ MEDITATION
- ☐ LOVING SELF-TALK
- ☐ DEEP BREATHING

RATE MY...

- ENERGY LEVEL ☆☆☆
- SELF-CARE ☆☆☆
- HUNGER/CRAVINGS ☆☆☆
- RELATIONSHIP WITH FOOD & EXERCISE ☆☆☆

ONE THING I WOULD LIKE TO KEEP WORKING ON _____

_____
_____

3 THINGS I AM GRATEFUL FOR TODAY

1. _____
2. _____
3. _____

# OF STEPS		% BODY FAT		WEIGHT	

Tuesday
WEEK 12

___/___/___

NUTRITION

	PROTEIN	STARCH	FRUIT	VEGETABLES	FATS
BREAKFAST 🕐					
MORNING SNACK 🕐					
LUNCH 🕐					
AFTERNOON SNACK 🕐					
DINNER 🕐					
EVENING SNACK 🕐					
TOTALS					

WATER 🍋 ② ③ ④ ⑤ ⑥ ⑦ ⑧ ⊕ ⊕ ⊕ ⊕

OTHER BEVERAGES _____

SUPPLEMENTS/MEDICATIONS _____

DIGESTION/BOWEL MOVEMENTS _____

> "I AM STRONG BECAUSE I'VE BEEN WEAK.
> I AM FEARLESS BECAUSE I'VE BEEN AFRAID.
> I AM WISE BECAUSE I'VE BEEN FOOLISH."
> - UNKNOWN

WHAT WOULD MAKE TODAY GREAT?

1. _____
2. _____
3. _____

MINDFULNESS

HOW DO I FEEL TODAY? _____
_____
_____
_____

MY MOOD IS...

- ☐ HAPPY
- ☐ FOCUSED
- ☐ ENERGETIC
- ☐ EXCITED
- ☐ SAD
- ☐ TIRED
- ☐ ANXIOUS
- ☐ ANGRY

I PRACTICED...

- ☐ MEDITATION
- ☐ LOVING SELF-TALK
- ☐ DEEP BREATHING

FITNESS

EXERCISE _____
_____
_____
_____

RATE MY...

- ENERGY LEVEL ☆☆☆
- SELF-CARE ☆☆☆
- HUNGER/CRAVINGS ☆☆☆
- RELATIONSHIP WITH FOOD & EXERCISE ☆☆☆

ONE THING I WOULD LIKE TO KEEP WORKING ON _____
_____
_____

3 THINGS I AM GRATEFUL FOR TODAY

1. _____
2. _____
3. _____

# OF STEPS	% BODY FAT	WEIGHT

Wednesday __/__/__
WEEK 12

NUTRITION

	PROTEIN	STARCH	FRUIT	VEGETABLES	FATS
BREAKFAST 🕐					
MORNING SNACK 🕐					
LUNCH 🕐					
AFTERNOON SNACK 🕐					
DINNER 🕐					
EVENING SNACK 🕐					
TOTALS					

WATER 💧 ② ③ ④ ⑤ ⑥ ⑦ ⑧ ➕ ➕ ➕ ➕

OTHER BEVERAGES _____

SUPPLEMENTS/MEDICATIONS _____

DIGESTION/BOWEL MOVEMENTS _____

> "NOTHING GREAT WAS EVER ACHIEVED
> WITHOUT ENTHUSIASM."
> - RALPH WALDO EMERSON

WHAT WOULD MAKE TODAY GREAT?

1. _____
2. _____
3. _____

MINDFULNESS

HOW DO I FEEL TODAY? _____
_____
_____
_____

MY MOOD IS...

- ☐ HAPPY
- ☐ SAD
- ☐ FOCUSED
- ☐ TIRED
- ☐ ENERGETIC
- ☐ ANXIOUS
- ☐ EXCITED
- ☐ ANGRY

FITNESS

EXERCISE _____
_____
_____
_____

I PRACTICED...

- ☐ MEDITATION
- ☐ LOVING SELF-TALK
- ☐ DEEP BREATHING

RATE MY...

- ENERGY LEVEL ☆☆☆
- SELF-CARE ☆☆☆
- HUNGER/CRAVINGS ☆☆☆
- RELATIONSHIP WITH FOOD & EXERCISE ☆☆☆

ONE THING I WOULD LIKE TO KEEP WORKING ON _____
_____
_____

3 THINGS I AM GRATEFUL FOR TODAY

1. _____
2. _____
3. _____

| # OF STEPS | | % BODY FAT | | WEIGHT | |

Thursday
WEEK 12

___/___/___

NUTRITION

	PROTEIN	STARCH	FRUIT	VEGETABLES	FATS
BREAKFAST 🕐					
MORNING SNACK 🕐					
LUNCH 🕐					
AFTERNOON SNACK 🕐					
DINNER 🕐					
EVENING SNACK 🕐					
TOTALS					

WATER ✦ 2 3 4 5 6 7 8 ⊕ ⊕ ⊕ ⊕

OTHER BEVERAGES _____

SUPPLEMENTS/MEDICATIONS _____

DIGESTION/BOWEL MOVEMENTS _____

> "SUCCESS IS STUMBLING FROM FAILURE TO FAILURE WITH NO LOSS OF ENTHUSIASM."
> - WINSTON CHURCHILL

WHAT WOULD MAKE TODAY GREAT?

1. _____
2. _____
3. _____

MINDFULNESS

HOW DO I FEEL TODAY? _____
_____
_____
_____

MY MOOD IS...

- ☐ HAPPY
- ☐ FOCUSED
- ☐ ENERGETIC
- ☐ EXCITED
- ☐ SAD
- ☐ TIRED
- ☐ ANXIOUS
- ☐ ANGRY

FITNESS

EXERCISE _____
_____
_____
_____

I PRACTICED...

- ☐ MEDITATION
- ☐ LOVING SELF-TALK
- ☐ DEEP BREATHING

RATE MY...

- ENERGY LEVEL ☆☆☆
- SELF-CARE ☆☆☆
- HUNGER/CRAVINGS ☆☆☆
- RELATIONSHIP WITH FOOD & EXERCISE ☆☆☆

ONE THING I WOULD LIKE TO KEEP WORKING ON _____
_____
_____

3 THINGS I AM GRATEFUL FOR TODAY

1. _____
2. _____
3. _____

# OF STEPS	% BODY FAT	WEIGHT

Friday
WEEK 12

___/___/___

NUTRITION

	PROTEIN	STARCH	FRUIT	VEGETABLES	FATS
BREAKFAST 🕐					
MORNING SNACK 🕐					
LUNCH 🕐					
AFTERNOON SNACK 🕐					
DINNER 🕐					
EVENING SNACK 🕐					
TOTALS					

WATER 💧 ② ③ ④ ⑤ ⑥ ⑦ ⑧ ⊕ ⊕ ⊕ ⊕

OTHER BEVERAGES _____

SUPPLEMENTS/MEDICATIONS _____

DIGESTION/BOWEL MOVEMENTS _____

> "THE REWARD OF A THING WELL DONE IS
> HAVING DONE IT."
> - RALPH WALDO EMERSON

WHAT WOULD MAKE TODAY GREAT?

1. _____
2. _____
3. _____

MINDFULNESS

HOW DO I FEEL TODAY? _____
_____
_____
_____

MY MOOD IS...
- ☐ HAPPY   ☐ SAD
- ☐ FOCUSED   ☐ TIRED
- ☐ ENERGETIC   ☐ ANXIOUS
- ☐ EXCITED   ☐ ANGRY

FITNESS

EXERCISE _____
_____
_____
_____

I PRACTICED...
- ☐ MEDITATION
- ☐ LOVING SELF-TALK
- ☐ DEEP BREATHING

RATE MY...
- ENERGY LEVEL ☆ ☆ ☆
- SELF-CARE ☆ ☆ ☆
- HUNGER/CRAVINGS ☆ ☆ ☆
- RELATIONSHIP WITH FOOD & EXERCISE ☆ ☆ ☆

ONE THING I WOULD LIKE TO KEEP WORKING ON _____
_____
_____

3 THINGS I AM GRATEFUL FOR TODAY

1. _____
2. _____
3. _____

☐ RECORD BODY MEASUREMENTS | # OF STEPS ____ | % BODY FAT ____ | WEIGHT ____

saturday
WEEK 12

___/___/___

NUTRITION

		PROTEIN	STARCH	FRUIT	VEGETABLES	FATS
BREAKFAST 🕐						
MORNING SNACK 🕐						
LUNCH 🕐						
AFTERNOON SNACK 🕐						
DINNER 🕐						
EVENING SNACK 🕐						
TOTALS						

WATER 💧 ② ③ ④ ⑤ ⑥ ⑦ ⑧ ⊕ ⊕ ⊕ ⊕

OTHER BEVERAGES _____

SUPPLEMENTS/MEDICATIONS _____

DIGESTION/BOWEL MOVEMENTS _____

"WONDER IS THE BEGINNING OF WISDOM."
- GREEK PROVERB

WHAT WOULD MAKE TODAY GREAT?

1. _____
2. _____
3. _____

MINDFULNESS

HOW DO I FEEL TODAY? _____
_____
_____
_____

MY MOOD IS...

- ☐ HAPPY
- ☐ FOCUSED
- ☐ ENERGETIC
- ☐ EXCITED
- ☐ SAD
- ☐ TIRED
- ☐ ANXIOUS
- ☐ ANGRY

FITNESS

EXERCISE _____
_____
_____
_____

I PRACTICED...

- ☐ MEDITATION
- ☐ LOVING SELF-TALK
- ☐ DEEP BREATHING

RATE MY...

- ENERGY LEVEL ☆ ☆ ☆
- SELF-CARE ☆ ☆ ☆
- HUNGER/CRAVINGS ☆ ☆ ☆
- RELATIONSHIP WITH FOOD & EXERCISE ☆ ☆ ☆

ONE THING I WOULD LIKE TO KEEP WORKING ON _____
_____
_____

3 THINGS I AM GRATEFUL FOR TODAY

1. _____
2. _____
3. _____

# OF STEPS		% BODY FAT		WEIGHT	

Sunday

WEEK 12

___/___/___

NUTRITION

		PROTEIN	STARCH	FRUIT	VEGETABLES	FATS
BREAKFAST 🕐						
MORNING SNACK 🕐						
LUNCH 🕐						
AFTERNOON SNACK 🕐						
DINNER 🕐						
EVENING SNACK 🕐						
TOTALS						

WATER 🍋 ② ③ ④ ⑤ ⑥ ⑦ ⑧ ⊕ ⊕ ⊕ ⊕

OTHER BEVERAGES _____

SUPPLEMENTS/MEDICATIONS _____

DIGESTION/BOWEL MOVEMENTS _____

**ASK YOURSELF TODAY:
WHAT DO I LOVE ABOUT MYSELF?**

WHAT WOULD MAKE TODAY GREAT?

1. _____
2. _____
3. _____

MINDFULNESS

HOW DO I FEEL TODAY? _____
_____
_____
_____

MY MOOD IS...

- ☐ HAPPY
- ☐ SAD
- ☐ FOCUSED
- ☐ TIRED
- ☐ ENERGETIC
- ☐ ANXIOUS
- ☐ EXCITED
- ☐ ANGRY

I PRACTICED...

- ☐ MEDITATION
- ☐ LOVING SELF-TALK
- ☐ DEEP BREATHING

FITNESS

EXERCISE _____
_____
_____
_____

RATE MY...

- ENERGY LEVEL ★ ★ ★
- SELF-CARE ★ ★ ★
- HUNGER/CRAVINGS ★ ★ ★
- RELATIONSHIP WITH FOOD & EXERCISE ★ ★ ★

ONE THING I WOULD LIKE TO KEEP WORKING ON _____
_____
_____

3 THINGS I AM GRATEFUL FOR TODAY

1. _____
2. _____
3. _____

| # OF STEPS | | % BODY FAT | | WEIGHT | |

Progress

Weight

DATE	WEIGHT	TOTAL LOSS/GAIN	% BODY FAT	NOTE

Tracker

DATE	WEIGHT	TOTAL LOSS/GAIN	% BODY FAT	NOTE

Weight

DATE	WEIGHT	TOTAL LOSS/GAIN	% BODY FAT	NOTE

Tracker

DATE	WEIGHT	TOTAL LOSS/GAIN	% BODY FAT	NOTE

Body

GOAL WEIGHT	

	START	WEEK 2	LOST	WEEK 4	LOST
DATE					
PRESENT WEIGHT					
WRIST (over wristbone)					
UPPER ARM (largest part)					
NECK (middle of neck)					
UPPER CHEST (directly below armpits)					
CHEST (along bust)					
MIDDRIFF (along lowest rib)					
WAIST (along bellybutton)					
ABDOMEN (widest part of belly)					
HIPS (widest part)					
THIGHS (largest part)					
KNEES (above kneecap)					
CALF (largest part)					
INCHES LOST					
TOTAL INCHES LOST					
WEIGHT LOST					
TOTAL WEIGHT LOSS					

Measurements

TOTAL WEIGHT LOSS				TOTAL INCHES LOST			
WEEK 6	LOST	WEEK 8	LOST	WEEK 10	LOST	WEEK 12	LOST

Favorite

BREAKFAST

LUNCH

Meals

DINNER

SNACKS

FOR HEALTHY RECIPE INSPIRATION VISIT COACHINGBYJENNIFER.COM/RECIPES

Weekly

Notes

Weekly

Notes

Weekly

Notes

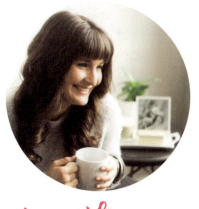

hey there!

My name is Jen and I am a Weight Loss and Lifestyle Coach and Personal Trainer with a passion for supporting others through the transformative journey of feeling more energetic, present, and comfortable in their bodies. Together, we create sustainable healthy habits and a sane and self-honoring approach to weight loss and lifetime weight management.

What makes me different from all the other coaches out there? Well, I've been there.

After struggling with excess weight, poor body image, compulsive eating, and yo-yo dieting throughout my adolescence and early 20's, I started my own journey towards creating sustainable changes in my own life, lost 70 pounds, and have been mindfully been exploring the journey of weight maintenance for the past ten years.

Since 2009, I have had the honor of supporting hundreds of others through their own transformation journeys through my signature nutrition, fitness, and lifestyle coaching programs.

While I grew up in the San Francisco Bay Area, I currently live in a row home in Philadelphia with my husband and son. When I'm not coaching, eating, or working out, I love reading, exploring the historical sites of Philly, and hosting rooftop BBQs.

Jennifer Lesyna Anthony
Certified Integrative Health Coach & Personal Trainer
Coaching by Jennifer | coachingbyjennifer.com

keep on working towards your goals!

CONGRATULATIONS ON ALL THE PROGRESS YOU HAVE MADE OVER THE LAST TWELVE WEEKS TOWARDS YOUR HEALTH AND WELLNESS GOALS.

I HOPE YOU'LL CONTINUE ON YOUR JOURNEY TO A HEALTHIER YOU BY ORDERING ANOTHER COPY OF THIS JOURNAL TO KEEP YOU INSPIRED AND ACCOUNTABLE!

ORDER ANOTHER COPY OF YOUR JOURNAL TODAY BY HEADING OVER TO COACHINGBYJENNIFER.COM/SHOP.

Jennifer Lesyna Anthony
Certified Integrative Health Coach & Personal Trainer
Coaching by Jennifer | coachingbyjennifer.com